Nutrition Relationships

Nutrition Relationships

**A PRACTICAL GUIDE TO DISCOVERING YOUR
UNIQUE NUTRITION NEEDS**

Jody Russ

2017

Nutrition Relationships

The content of this book is for general instruction only. Each person's physical, emotional, and spiritual condition is unique. The instruction in this book is not intended to replace or interrupt the reader's relationship with a physician or other professional. Please consult your doctor for matters pertaining to your specific health and diet.

To contact the publisher, visit
WEBSITE

To contact the author, email: sargeinshape@gmail.com

ISBN-13: **9781537577012**
ISBN-10: **1537577018**
Library of Congress Control Number: 2016915294
CreateSpace Independent Publishing Platform
North Charleston, South Carolina
Printed in the United States of America

Table of Contents

Introduction

'm convinced that food is the ultimate answer to our physical, mental, and social well-being. No matter your station or what endeavor of life you are in, energy is the one constant that makes or breaks us. And unless someone has found something other than food to energize us, we are stuck with food as our major source. If we are to be as healthy and as well as we can be, our food has to play a major role. If you have heard this before, it is worth hearing again, and if you have never heard this, welcome to the real world. You become healthy from the inside out. No amount of physical activity can overcome bad nutrition. Even in relationships the physical attraction will fade much faster than the mental and emotional attraction. We love our favorite restaurants because of the food that is prepared inside, not the beauty of the building. No other resource has contributed or detracted from my overall quality of life than my nutrition. Not money, not notoriety, not life accomplishments. Add what you will to the list. If you are constantly physically sick, stressed out, overweight, underweight, diabetic—again, add what you will to the list—no amount of money, fame, or fortune will improve your quality of life. I searched the Internet and found there were over 270 shows about food on TV. Time would not allow me to research how many cookbooks have been published or restaurants opened.

First and foremost, we need food for survival. I know that is stating the obvious, but it is worth repeating. Food heals us. Food makes us sick. Food comforts us. Food has become our friend when we are lonely. In some cases food has become our enemy through bulimia and other unhealthy diet trends. Food defines us as cultures. Food makes us money as well as loses us money. Food is a platform for political debate. Food has been the cause of addiction. Food has caused stress through allergies. I could go on a while longer, but you get the point. Food is everything to most people. Whether we want to accept it or not, we all have a lifelong love affair with food. In the preceding statements, you can replace the word "food" with a person, whoever that person may be. I would like to take the stance that we treat our food as a person whom we are married to for life. This marriage is not one of convenience but one of necessity. This is the mate you cannot live without, and he or she will have a major impact on your physical, mental, emotional, and authentic self until death do you part.

I sincerely believe that one of the most misunderstood concepts in a relationship is the lack of self-awareness. Furthermore, I believe most unions fail because of lack of communication. This supports the concept of self-awareness. You have to know who you are and what makes you tick before you can even begin to connect with a partner. If you don't cover this ground first, you leave it to the other person to define you. And that is a very slippery slope for survival. I use the term "survive" because your life will be a constant game of who am I. In this book we will explore the intimate relationship we have with food. You will see that just as in any relationship, you must take control of the relationship in terms of what is good and bad for you. This journey will be laced with science-based, real-world relationship connections that will help you manage this phenomenon that has plagued our health and well-being for centuries.

You will see that once you reach a level of relationship health with this life force, your vision of real wellness will become clear. Like a parent who knows his or her child, you will be able to nurture your relationship with food, and it will respect and serve you well for the rest of your life. I hope you are ready to engage in a lifelong, fulfilling, and meaningful relationship.

CHAPTER 1

Knowing Yourself

In this chapter we explore these elements:

- your beginnings
- your basic survival needs
- your initial genetic blueprint

This may seem like an easy task to most. "I've known myself my whole life, and I think I'm the authority on any and everything pertaining to me," most will proclaim. But, as I tell my students, sometimes we get a better understanding of the vehicle if we consult the manufacturer, namely your parents. Our manufacturer is always in question by society. You either believe in creation or evolution. I'm not even going to try to take a side on that. Let's just agree that medical science is our manufacturer. It doesn't take into account either belief from the standpoint of what makes us tick. And most people tend to put great faith in science, for the most part. It is a common truth that our bodies need calories (the energy needed to raise the temperature of 1 gram of water through 1°C) to continuously perform any task. The issue becomes how many and what kind we need. First, let me insult your intelligence for a little while. Everything we eat has some form of calories. But all calories are not created equal. Just like gasoline to the car, there are low- and high-grade calories. Now, because I know we are intelligent beings, I don't have to explain too much. But here we go.

We basically survive and get our energy through photosynthesis, as we all know. Now it would be nice if we could just walk outside and absorb all the energy we need and be done with it. Our systems don't work that way. But just in case you were not paying attention in science class, photosynthesis is a process used by plants and other organisms to convert light energy, normally from the sun, into chemical energy that can be later released to fuel our activities. During photosynthesis, light energy is absorbed in plant cells and converted with carbon dioxide (from the air) and water (from the soil) into a sugar called glucose. Oxygen is released as a by-product. When that light hits your cells, it releases an electron that generates the energy needed to power your cells for work. This energy, once again, is called glucose. We will explore this source in detail later. Now, that is the *Reader's Digest* version, but you get the picture. From an ecological standpoint, this is why plants are so important to our existence. So basically, we are at our core are plants when it comes to our survival. Just keep us in the sun for a little bit and give us some water, the occasional ingestion of plants, maybe some meat for variety, a little activity, and we will live to be one hundred years old. OK, have a nice life. Now, I know this is going to sound a little crazy to those of us who are not plant people, as I am in that number. There are people out there who actually talk to and have real relationships with their plants and animals. Believe it or not, they are not crazy in the least bit. They have probably lived enough life to get fed up with humans and see the true benefit of genuine friendship with something that shows unconditional love. I'm not there quite yet. Interaction is also a part of who we are. No man or woman is an island. So we are left oftentimes to our relationships and circumstances to complete the blueprint of who we are and what we will become. So let's now explore this second aspect of knowing ourselves—the family reunion.

A nice trip to the family reunion should do the trick. Look around and take note of certain things: body types, ages, habits, attitudes, and any other statistic that you decide is important to the identification of you. Don't be alarmed at things you may not like or approve of. Yes, everyone has the intoxicated uncle, annoying cousin, or hug-thirsty aunt. Embrace the history and culture that has created you. This will give you some insight into who you are or why you do certain things or act a certain way. This is your origin. This is your photosynthesis, your interaction code, your water, and other macro/micro nutrient profile. In many recipes there are certain ingredients that you would not eat alone, but in conjunction with the finished product, they become valuable components of the entire experience. Just as there are certain foods or practices that are not healthful for your body, there are things you will find out or people you will meet at the family reunion who are not healthful for your mental or emotional health. But it is better to know and build strategies to help you cope with or eliminate those whom you can. I believe you can become more in control of your destiny and be a more well-adjusted partner in any relationship. As we have heard so many times past, those who ignore history are bound to repeat it. Now, some history is good and some bad. It is best to get the truth, the whole truth, and nothing but the truth. This trip to the family reunion in no way is the final determining factor as to what we become. So don't become depressed or develop low self-esteem over what you perceive is the negative side of your blueprint. This could be a blessing in disguise. On the other hand, don't think you have it made because you like what you see. You still have work to do. We use the past to give us information to change or somewhat modify the future for the better. There are even people who have become famous for revealing what they see at family reunions. They are called comedians. So take a light-hearted view of what you see at your blueprint gathering. Humor is stress relieving and healthy. Armed with this information, and maybe therapy for some of us, we can begin to know what we need to be our best selves and navigate our relationships in a healthy and balanced manner.

In summary: Know your history. Embrace your history, the good and the bad. Understand where you came from. It is the foundation or framework for your ultimate purpose. It will help you answer many questions about what motivates you, challenges you, and fulfills you, and it will answer other specific questions about your existence. Understand where you get your energy from. It will be your source of strength to be as healthy and well as you can be. We have just scratched the surface when it comes to building a solid and healthy relationship with our food. Now let's get more personal with our needs.

CHAPTER 2

Knowing What Everyone Basically Needs

In this chapter we explore:

- The glucose phenomenon
- Properties of the major macronutrients
- The superpower of water
- Suggested quantities of nutrient consumption
- Strategy for weight maintenance

I put the term "basically" in the title of this chapter because just as you cannot write a sentence without knowing words first, you must know basic nutrition before you can give yourself what you individually need. Here is a philosophy I have found that takes the guesswork out of what you should or should not eat. We are living things, and our bodies recognize living things. So if you ingest anything living, your body has very little problem processing it unless you have some type of metabolic dysfunction or the living thing is in some way contaminated. So if it grows from the ground (plants) or had parents (animals), I believe it will give your body what it needs to be strong and well if you eat it as close to its natural state as possible. I know that is going to kick-start all kinds of debate over not eating or eating this or that being right or wrong. Make your own judgment.

Before any decisions can be made about what you need, a trip to the doctor is a good first step. The doctor can let you know if there are any unhealthy physiological or chemical issues with you. But, believe it or not, doctors are not trained extensively in nutrition, so that is only part of your starting point. Relationship wise, your doctor is that person or mentor you know who is at least a generation older than you and has lived enough life to give you life-experience advice. It could be a parent, teacher, or other family member whom you trust. Just as doctors aren't fully trained in nutrition, your mentor is not growing up in your generation, and the relationship game, just like nutrition, changes over time. The mentor could probably give advice from a personal and emotional perspective, possibly coloring the advice given. So take all advice with a grain of sodium, but not too much, and continue reading.

From the preceding information, it is apparent we need plants. So it should go without saying that we need to eat plants for basic energy and survival. But I will say it anyway. "We need to eat plants for basic energy and survival." I will hold the discussion on the need for fats, proteins, and other vitamins and minerals for later because our need for them (quality and quantity) is dependent on so many factors other than basic survival. Now we can finish the glucose story. The name **glucose** is from the Greek word for "sweet." Glucose is a **monosaccharide**, which is another term for a simple sugar. It is one of three monosaccharides that are used by the body, but it is the only one that can be used directly to produce human energy. Thus, adequate glucose levels are essential. As mentioned, glucose is used by cells to make energy and power the body.

Relationship Perspective: In a relationship, our glucose is considered our energy. If I have learned anything in life, it's that energy is a large component of any endeavor, specifically in relationships. We don't normally consider it energy until it becomes a problem. That is why many feel that living together before getting married is a smart move. You get a chance to sample the energy exchange with your partner. I will not judge on that concept. But I will say the fall of many unions can be traced back to competing or unbalanced energy sources. The term commonly used is that we just "grew apart" or our goals "did not align." Now let's discuss the types of energy that are on the market and available for purchase.

My knowledge from the Institute of Integrative Nutrition® drives in the direction of using food for fuel first and enjoyment second. This means it is more beneficial to view our intake as energy for work and/or play. If we shift our intake focus in this direction, we will mentally condition ourselves to look for the best energy we can find. In a relationship, unless you are psychic, you don't see the energy of the person you desire. We generally get caught up in the outer appearance or the wrapping paper of the gift. If you are looking at other qualities in a mate, you are way ahead of the game in long-term happiness and fulfillment. So let's explore beyond the nice locks of hair, white teeth, contact-infused eyes, beach-perfect body, and captivating conversation.

It is not the intent of this book to advocate any specific diet as the supreme law of the land. And is it just me, or are the first letters of the word "diet" a little unsettling? I believe whatever diet or style of eating you have has good and bad effects. We are all individuals and respond to certain stimuli in different ways. No two humans are genetically identical. Genes and environment influence human biological variation, from visible characteristics to physiology to disease susceptibly to mental abilities. The exact influence of genes and environment on certain traits is not well understood.

The human body's ability to adapt to different environmental stresses is remarkable, allowing humans to acclimatize to a wide range of temperatures, humidity, and altitudes.

The field of nutrition is ever changing, and new protocols and knowledge about all facets of food are in constant flux. In the interests of education, let's talk about what was never, is not now, nor will never be in flux—our macronutrients.

Carbohydrates

Our systems are energized most efficiently by the quality in our nutritional relationship with the energy known as carbohydrates. They give us four calories per gram but provide many more benefits than just energy. There are two varieties of carbohydrates.

The Simple Carbohydrates

Let's just call simple carbohydrates infatuation—the I-want-it-right-now kind of energy. Simple carbohydrates are broken down quickly by the body to be used as energy. There is good simple and bad simple.

First, the good. Good carbohydrates are found naturally in foods. Tell me, have you ever seen these things growing in a garden, on a tree, or in a field, or come from living things?

- Fruit
- Milk
- Milk products

Of course you have. The key word in these sugars is "natural," which means the sugar was part of the organism from birth if it was an animal or from the ground if it grew.

Less processing from the origin of a food product to consumption yields more benefit from the food product. Not only do you get the sweet taste, you get vitamins and minerals for healthy bones, muscles, immune system, and nerve function, just to name a few. You also get fiber from the plant products, which assists in digestion and slowing the rise in blood sugar. As Hippocrates, the famous Greek physician, said, "Let food be thy medicine."

Relationship perspective: Our good simple carbohydrates are our lifelong friends that have always been there for us, but a long-term, committed relationship just wouldn't work. We know this from experience, but we still enjoy their presence for the moment and then go our separate ways.

And now, the bad. These simple carbohydrates have been processed and refined and do not resemble the origin of the organism. Tell me, have you ever seen these things growing in a garden, on a tree, or in a field, or come from a living thing?

- Candy
- Table Sugar
- Syrups
- Soft Drinks
- Pastries

No, you have not. They do not have the vitamins, minerals, and fiber that your body recognizes and can process easily. What you get is a quick, natural high and sweet taste from the sugar; an insulin surge without the fiber to slow the sugar; and, finally, the crash to your system as it tries to recover from the foreign materials ingested. High-grade inflammation, which will be discussed later, diabetes, and heart disease are just a few of the energy-depleting and life-threatening results.

Relationship perspective: Picture the bad boy or bad girl who you think would up your street cred or bad reputation for a while. You know going in that it's probably an accident waiting happen, but man, it would feel great to have that on your resume. What ensues is eventual low self-esteem, weight gain, lack of energy, lack of sleep, and overall depression, among other mental and social abnormalities. You see, the simple sugars don't have time to hang around and attend to you. They have other clients just waiting. Some of us can recognize them at events from their conversation. You know:

"Your feet must be tired because you've been running through my mind all night." Or "Heaven must be missing an angel." The female simple sugar is a little subtler. You know: dancing a little more seductively than everyone else, or the more up-front "Can you buy me a drink?" We need to minimize or at best cut off these types of relationships. Or maybe you like that type of sugar and what it could possibly bring to the table.

And Now, Complex Carbohydrates

We can consider complex carbohydrates mid- to high-grade fuel. Complex carbohydrates may be referred to as dietary starch and are made of sugar molecules strung together like a necklace or branched like a coil. They are often rich in fiber; thus, they're satisfying and health promoting. Complex carbohydrates are commonly found in whole plant foods and therefore are also often high in vitamins and minerals. Tell me, have you ever seen these things growing in a garden, on a tree, or in a field, or come from a living thing?

- Green vegetables
- Whole grains and foods made from them, such as oatmeal, pasta, and whole-grain breads
- Starchy vegetables such as potatoes, sweet potatoes, corn, and pumpkins
- Beans, lentils, and peas

Of course you have.

Relationship Perspective: Picture your best friend from childhood, whom you have kept in contact with. It doesn't matter what stage of life you go through; you can depend on that friend to be there for you—comforting you, laughing with you, having the guts to be brutally honest with you when you need it, and being your lifelong confidant. These people are your complex carbohydrates. They give you energy and help balance you physically, mentally, and emotionally. Have you ever fallen out of good grace with one of these friends? You feel very uncomfortable and could become physically sick, lose sleep, and become very unproductive until you make it right with that true friend. That person has been there for you from the beginning. Value that relationship. For another perspective, consider the married couple that has been together twenty years with minimal problems or distractions from a relationship perspective.

This is a relationship rich in fiber and consistency. The kids are now grown and have moved out, and they're beginning to seek other sources of fulfillment. The marriage is now in a state of dysfunction because the fiber has been replaced by other interests.

Fats

First let me say that fat has been given a bad reputation for contributing to poor health. There are numerous types of fat. Your body makes its own fat from taking in excess calories. Some fats are found in foods from plants and animals and are known as dietary fat. Just like most things in a nutrition relationship, there are good and bad aspects of this quality.

Helpful Dietary Fats

Let's check the good qualities first. These types of potentially helpful dietary fat are mostly unsaturated:

Monounsaturated fatty acids. These fats are liquid at room temperature and solid when chilled. Monounsaturated fats are typically high in vitamin E, which is a vitamin that Americans tend to need. Common monounsaturated fats are oils, nuts, seeds, fish, cheese, and, I will add for the sake of satisfaction, dark chocolate.

Polyunsaturated fatty acids. At the risk of repeating myself, these fats are similar to the mono type, with the exception that their chemical bond is a little stronger. Sorry for that bit of chemistry. It was necessary. The examples are basically the same.

Omega-3 fatty acids. Omega-3s are "essential" fatty acids because the body isn't capable of producing them on its own. Therefore, we must rely on omega-3 foods in our diet to supply these extremely beneficial compounds. The preferred sources are seafood such as salmon and sardines. They are also found in some plant foods, including certain nuts and seeds, as well as high-quality cuts of meat such as grass-fed beef. Historically, we've seen that the populations that consume the most omega-3 foods, such as people in Okinawa, Japan, live longer and healthier lives than people who eat a standard diet low in omega-3s. The typical Okinawa diet—which consists of plenty of fish, sea vegetables, and other fresh produce—is actually believed to have about eight times the amount of omega-3s that you'd find in the standard American diet, which is likely one reason why this population is considered one of the healthiest in human history.

So, as you can see, all the bad things you have been hearing about fat you shouldn't put too much weight on. I know, pardon the pun. Here is a list of things the good fat does for your health:

Organ protection: Obviously, our bodies and organs are protected with a reasonable portion of fat.

Digestion: Fat dissolves in blood so it can store critical vitamins A, D, E, and K in the liver and fatty tissues. It also keeps you satisfied.

Transport: Fat is a part of every cell membrane in your body. It helps transport nutrients across cell membranes.

Conversion: Your body utilizes fat for everything from activating hormones to building immune function.

Energy extraction: Between meals and when glucose is not available, fats are broken down for energy, which, in times of great need, the brain's neurons can use.

Nervous system: Fat is 80 percent of the protective coating of nerves.

But fat is high in calories—nine calories per gram. If you eat more calories than you need, you will gain weight. Excess weight is linked to poor health. In addition, some types of dietary fat are thought to play a role in cardiovascular disease. Research about the possible harms and benefits of dietary fat is always evolving. And a growing body of research suggests that when it comes to dietary fat, you should focus on eating healthy fats and avoiding unhealthy fats.

Harmful Dietary Fats

Harmful dietary fats raise total blood cholesterol levels and low-density lipoprotein (LDL) cholesterol levels and increase your risk of cardiovascular disease and type 2 diabetes. There are two main types of potentially harmful dietary fat:

Saturated Fat: Saturated fats are typically solid at room temperature. Saturated fats occur naturally in many foods. The majority come mainly from animal sources, including meat and dairy products. Some examples are:

- fatty beef
- lamb
- pork
- poultry with skin
- beef fat (tallow)
- lard and cream
- butter
- cheese and other dairy products made from whole or reduced-fat (2 percent) milk

In addition, many baked goods and fried foods can contain high levels of saturated fats. Some plant-based oils, such as palm oil, palm kernel oil, and coconut oil also contain primarily saturated fats, but they do not contain cholesterol.

Eating foods that contain saturated fats raises the level of cholesterol in your blood. High levels of LDL cholesterol in your blood increase your risk of heart disease and stroke.

Trans fat: There are two broad types of trans fats found in foods: naturally occurring and artificial trans fats.

Naturally occurring trans fats are produced in the gut of some animals, and foods made from these animals (e.g., milk and meat products) may contain small quantities of these fats.

Artificial trans fats are created in an industrial process that adds hydrogen to liquid vegetable oils to make them more solid.

Trans fats are easy to use, inexpensive to produce, and last a long time. Trans fats give foods a desirable taste and texture. Many restaurants and fast-food outlets use trans fats to deep fry foods because oils with trans fats can be used many times in commercial fryers. Trans fats can be found in many foods, including:

- fried foods such as doughnuts

- baked goods, including:
  - cakes
  - pie crusts
  - biscuits
  - frozen pizza
  - cookies

- ○ crackers
- ○ stick margarines and other spreads.

Trans fats raise your bad (LDL) cholesterol levels and lower your good (HDL) cholesterol levels. Eating trans fats increases your risk of developing heart disease and stroke. It's also associated with a higher risk of developing type 2 diabetes. The American Heart Association recommends that adults who would benefit from lowering LDL cholesterol reduce their intake of trans fat and limit their consumption of saturated fat to 5 to 6 percent of total calories.

Here are some ways to achieve that:

- Eat a dietary pattern that emphasizes fruits, vegetables, whole grains, low-fat dairy products, poultry, fish, and nuts. Also limit red meat and sugary foods and beverages.
- Use naturally occurring, unhydrogenated vegetable oils such as canola, safflower, sunflower, or olive oil most often.
- Look for processed foods made with unhydrogenated oil rather than partially hydrogenated or hydrogenated vegetable oils or saturated fat.
- Use margarine as a substitute for butter, and choose soft margarines (liquid or tub varieties) over harder stick forms. Look for "0 g trans fat" on the Nutrition Facts label and no hydrogenated oils in the ingredients list.
- Doughnuts, cookies, crackers, muffins, pies, and cakes are examples of foods that may contain trans fat. Limit how frequently you eat them.
- Limit commercially fried foods and baked goods made with shortening or partially hydrogenated vegetable oils. Not only are these foods very high in fat, but that fat is also likely to be trans fat.

Relationship Perspective: Our good fats are friends that we need for specific purposes. They make us laugh, but we don't want to laugh all the time. They are very serious, but we don't want to be serious all the time. They are very emotional, but we don't want to be emotional all the time. The list could go on and on. Bottom line, they are essential to our total well-being in moderation. But they do carry nine calories per gram, so they can become heavy if we don't utilize some restraint. He is heavy, and he's our brother—look up the song, my younger readers. On the other hand, our bad fats are those friends that have fallen in with wrong crowd, joined gangs, or have somehow lost their way. They are either criminals or well on their way to hard lives.

We hardly even recognize them. They have been heavily processed through a system we know very little about, and if we try to save them, we will be guilty by association and possibly suffer the same or similar fate. It is best we leave them alone. Let the authorities deal with them. Maybe they will survive, and we will be able to recognize them in another life.

Protein

Proteins are large, complex molecules that play many critical roles in the body. They do most of the work in cells and are required for the structure, function, and regulation of the body's tissues and organs. Proteins are made up of hundreds of thousands of smaller units called amino acids, which are attached to one another in long chains. There are twenty different types of amino acids that can be combined to make a protein. The sequence of amino acids determines each protein's unique three-dimensional structure and its specific function. Proteins can be described according to their large range of functions in the body. Protein is an important component of every cell in the body. Hair and nails are mostly made of protein. Your body uses protein to build and repair tissues. You also use protein to make enzymes, hormones, and other body chemicals. Protein is an important building block of bones, muscles, cartilage, skin, and blood.

Here are ten terrific sources of lean protein:

- Fish
- Seafood
- Skinless white-meat poultry
- Lean beef (including tenderloin, sirloin, eye of round)
- Skim or low-fat milk
- Skim or low-fat yogurt
- Fat-free or low-fat cheese
- Eggs
- Lean pork (tenderloin)
- Beans

Relationship Perspective: Protein is your parents, grandparents, aunts, uncles, or any other adult who had the pleasure of being in the village that raised you. Yes, I said it.

Our village knows us better than anyone. Our parents gave us the protein we have. They know things about us that we don't know about ourselves. Protein builds strong bodies and repairs damaged tissues. Isn't that basically what our village did for us? We may not like the advice, but they normally speak from experience. Now, don't get me wrong; I know there are a few villages out there that have some very poor builders for whatever reason. Those are the ones that have a lot of fat left on the meat. Sometimes we have to cut the fat away.

Water

In general, humans can survive for two to eight weeks without food, depending on stored body fat. Survival without water is usually limited to three or four days. About thirty-six million humans die every year from causes directly or indirectly related to hunger.

The human body contains from 55 to 78 percent water, depending on body size. To function properly, the body requires between one and seven liters of water per day to avoid dehydration; the precise amount depends on the level of activity, temperature, humidity, and other factors. Most of this is ingested through foods or beverages other than drinking straight water. It is not clear how much water intake healthy people need, though most specialists agree that approximately two liters (six to seven glasses) of water daily is the minimum to maintain proper hydration. Medical literature favors a lower consumption, typically one liter of water for an average male, excluding extra requirements due to fluid loss from exercise or warm weather.

Relationship perspective: Water is the one element in our life that, no matter what we are going through, brings us peace and comfort. It is not a person, because people change. Water is constant, always giving us what we need at the moment. It is cleansing and refreshing. It is that me-time activity that always brings us back to center. My water is art, music, and fitness. It doesn't have to involve a person. Sometimes adding a person adds drama. I know I have a few witnesses on that one. What is your water? Reading? Meditation? Hiking? Fishing? There is no substitute for our water. If you let a person become your water, that person controls your center and therefore your true happiness.

As you can see, we as humans need many energy sources and maintenance support just to survive, let alone thrive. So the burning question for most of us is, how much of each quality do *I* need for optimum functioning? I emphasize the "I" because it is an individual thing. It is what we in the Integrative Nutrition® world refer to as bio individuality. The goal in bioindividuality is to find out what is considered the perfect storm for each individual to thrive and be as well as he or she can.

Relationship perspective: It is finding that partner who has what can be considered the total package. For some it is a nice body, good conversation, and a strong religious conviction. For others it is financial stability, a good sense of humor, and a high level of education. It could be a combination of all or none of the above. It is what makes us happy. There is no one size that fits all packages on the market. There are a few constants that are needed for basic survival, but even those are negotiable to a certain extent. We need money, but how much is negotiable, depending on the person. We need a home and possibly transportation, but what kind and how new or old is negotiable, depending on the person. Nutritionally, everyone needs fats, carbohydrates, proteins, vitamins, and minerals. How much of each depends on gender, genetic profile, environment, social interaction, disease susceptibility, and a host of other factors that could take center stage.

Just as a point of reference, here is what the USDA recommends:

Fats: Keep total intake between 20 and 35 percent of calories, with most coming from sources of polyunsaturated and monounsaturated fatty acids, such as fish, nuts, and vegetable oils.

Carbohydrates: Keep total intake between 45 and 65 percent of calories, with most coming from fiber-rich fruits, vegetables, and whole grains. Choose and prepare foods and beverages with little added sugars or caloric sweeteners.

Protein: Keep total intake between 10 and 35 percent of calories, with most coming from animal sources, such as meat, poultry, fish, eggs, milk, cheese, and yogurt. Proteins from plants, legumes, grains, nuts, seeds, and vegetables tend to be deficient in one or more of the indispensable amino acids and are called "incomplete proteins."

Sodium: Consume less than 2,300 milligrams of sodium per day (approximately one teaspoon of salt). Choose and prepare foods with little salt. At the same time, consume potassium-rich foods such as fruits and vegetables.

Sugar: Men should consume less than 150 calories per day (37.5 grams or 9 teaspoons) and women less than 100 calories per day (25 grams or 6 teaspoons) of added sugars.

Alcoholic Beverages: Alcohol may have beneficial effects on chronic disease risk when consumed in moderation. However, heavy alcohol consumption increases risk for liver disease, high blood pressure, and certain cancers. Some people should avoid alcohol completely.

Obviously there are many more substances we need to be as healthy as we can, but these are the major players that contribute the most to overall wellness. Pay close attention that these are just recommendations. Because we all have some differences on a cellular and genetic level, you will have to find what works for your specific makeup. One person's medicine could be another person's poison. What makes one person happy in a relationship may bring conflict in another. There is no one size fits all when it comes to most things.

Here is a proven biological concept from my personal training experience that gives a baseline for nutritional needs from a weight-management perspective. If you multiply your weight by ten, that is the lowest number of calories you need to just exist. When I say "just exist," I mean no extra movement—just heart beating, breathing, the occasional trip to the restroom, and so on. The more we move, the more calories we will burn. For instance, a 180-pound person will need 1,800 calories just to survive. Of those 1,800 calories, it is up to your own bioindividuality how many fats and carbohydrates and how much protein you need to operate at optimal efficiency. We could go by the standard that the USDA recommends, but that wouldn't apply to everybody because everyone's genetic makeup is different. The only information I will leave you with for consumption of your fuel is to try to get the most of your fuel intake from complex carbohydrates and protein and less from the fats category, and drink plenty of water. Now, that is a healthy relationship.

Here is another little tidbit of information that is so simple that most people tend to not consider it. If our goal is to lose weight, it stands to reason that whatever our diet and activity level is right now is keeping us at that weight. So everyone has a baseline to start with from a fuel-intake perspective. And, to quote an old saying, "The definition of insanity is doing the same thing and expecting a different result."

One last nugget of knowledge that most people tend to oversimplify is that to eat less means to weigh less. There are so many other factors that influence this phenomenon. Loss of body weight depends highly on how your body burns the fuel you give it, which is called your metabolism. Less fuel means fewer logs on the metabolic furnace, causing your metabolism to slow down and store fat for future energy needs. It is a throwback from prehistoric times. So we need more of the right quality and quantity of energy, combined with healthy activity, for the best weight management and health. If we give the body what it needs, it will take care of the rest.

Let me introduce you to a friend of mine who could be a pretty good mate for you. He or she has all the good qualities any person could really need, not necessarily want. He or she is very attractive, has good morals and a great sense of humor, is physically fit, and has great conversation. I could go on, but I know the suspense is killing you. It is our integrative nutrition plate:

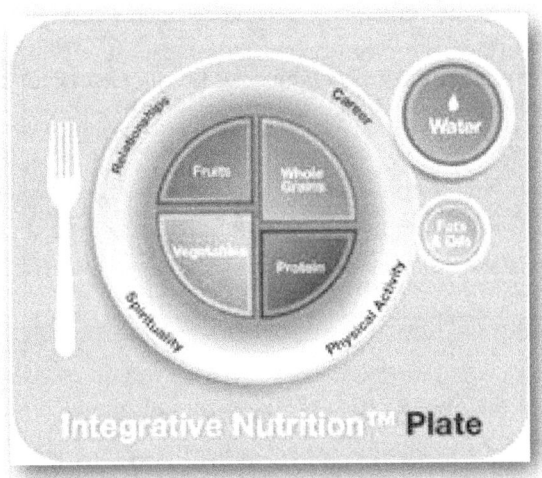

Integrative Nutrition® Plate

If you look closely, you will see the right amount of all the good qualities you need. Around the edges of the plate you see relationships, career, spirituality, and physical activity. You see all these aspects of life feed us all in the sense that they either give us energy or take it away from us. So it is important that we look at them as food. In Integrative Nutrition®, these are considered primary foods. They constantly feed us at a rate that far exceeds the natural foods. So we must give these energy sources some consideration. If either one of these energy sources is out of balance with your true self, then you are not living up to your true potential.

Here are a few tips on managing healthy eating:

Ensure you start the day with a healthy breakfast consisting of complex carbohydrates, protein, healthy fats, and water.

Stay hydrated throughout the day.

Bring your food or snacks with you so you know what you're consuming and not leaving it to others to decide.

Eat at least three meals and three or four small, healthy snacks a day to keep your metabolism burning. A meal can be a piece of cheese with almonds or a celery stick with peanut butter.

Ensure you are eating some form of protein with each meal. It is satisfying and builds muscle, which in turn burns fat.

Stay active throughout the day to keep muscles burning fat, which assists with digestion also.

I am by no means a chef or the least bit qualified to give any professional advice on cooking. But there are certain healthy ways of preparing food that yields the most benefit. Here are just a few:

Healthy cooking

- Stock up on heart-healthy cookbooks and recipes for cooking ideas.
- Use choice or select grades of beef rather than prime, and be sure to trim the fat off the edges before cooking.
- Use cuts of red meat and pork labeled "loin" and "round," as they usually have the least fat.
- With poultry, use the leaner light meat (breasts) instead of the fattier dark meat (legs and thighs), and be sure to remove the skin.
- Make recipes or egg dishes with egg whites instead of egg yolks. Substitute two egg whites for each egg yolk.
- For recipes that require dairy products, try low-fat or fat-free versions of milk, yogurt, and cheese.
- Use reduced-fat, low-fat, light, or no-fat salad dressings (if you need to limit your calories) on salads, for dips, or as marinades.
- Use and prepare foods that contain little or no salt.

Seasonings

- Avoid using prepackaged seasoning mixes because they often contain a lot of salt. Use fresh herbs whenever possible. Grind herbs with a mortar and pestle for the freshest and fullest flavor.

- Add dried herbs such as thyme, rosemary, and marjoram to dishes for a more pungent flavor—but use them sparingly because they're powerful.
- Use vinegar or citrus juice as wonderful flavor enhancers—but add them at the last moment. Vinegar is great on vegetables such as greens, and citrus works well on fruits such as melons.
- Use dry mustard for a zesty flavor when you're cooking, or mix it with water to make a very sharp condiment.
- To add a little more "bite" to your dishes, add some fresh hot peppers. Remove the membrane and seeds first and then finely chop them up. A small amount goes a long way.
- Some vegetables and fruits, such as mushrooms, tomatoes, chili peppers, cherries, cranberries, and currants, have a more intense flavor when dried than when fresh. Add them when you want a burst of flavor.

Oils

- Use liquid vegetable oils or nonfat cooking sprays whenever possible.
- Whether cooking or making dressings, use the oils that are lowest in saturated fats, trans fats, and cholesterol—such as canola oil, corn oil, olive oil, safflower oil, sesame oil, soybean oil, and sunflower oil—but use them sparingly, because they contain 120 calories per tablespoon.
- Stay away from coconut oil, palm oil, and palm kernel oil. Even though they are vegetable oils and have no cholesterol, they are high in saturated fats.

Instead of frying foods—which adds unnecessary fats and calories—use cooking methods that add little or no fat, such as these:

- **Stir-frying.** Use a wok to cook vegetables, poultry, or seafood in vegetable stock, wine, or a small amount of oil. Avoid high-sodium (salt) seasonings such as teriyaki and soy sauce.
- **Roasting.** Use a rack in the pan so the meat or poultry doesn't sit in its own fat drippings. Instead of basting with pan drippings, use fat-free liquids such as wine, tomato juice, or lemon juice. When making gravy from the drippings, chill first and then use a gravy strainer or skimming ladle to remove the fat.
- **Grilling and broiling.** Use a rack so the fat drips away from the food.
- **Baking.** Bake foods in covered cookware with a little extra liquid.

- **Poaching.** Cook chicken or fish by immersing it in simmering liquid.
- **Sautéing.** Use a pan made with nonstick metal or a coated, nonstick surface so you will need to use little or no oil when cooking. Use a nonstick vegetable spray to brown or sauté foods, or, as an alternative, use a small amount of broth or wine or a tiny bit of vegetable oil rubbed onto the pan with a paper towel.
- **Steaming.** Steam vegetables in a basket over simmering water. They'll retain more flavors and won't need any salt.

One final note about the condition of your food. From a relationship perspective it has already been established that you should know your partner. If you raised a child, you know more about that child from a behavior perspective because you shaped and engineered the organism. It is also good to know the background and associations of people you plan to enter into a relationship with. It is just good relationship etiquette. Unless you have been living under a rock for the past 30 years you have heard the term organic in every aspect of food from preparation to overall handling. Organic is defined as relating to or derived from living matter. From a food perspective it basically means the food did not have pesticides or other unnatural additives if it is a plant or was not injected with foreign substances if is an animal. It is how the organism was raised. It is scientifically proven that organic is healthier than non-organic. I will not attempt to explain the finer details of organic food.

http://www.sustainablefood.com/guide/orglinks.html has great information on the subject. You will find that organic will cost a little more. I believe it is a matter of personal preference and financial necessity and not an overall health necessity to choose organic. Once again I feel that bio-individuality dictates unless there are other health related issues identified by a medical professional. As always listen to your doctor.

Summary: It is so important that we understand the inner workings of our primary system of energy. We are living creatures that thrive on living things as close to their origin as possible. Once we get a report card from the doctor, we can begin our journey toward real health and wellness. Consume only the highest-quality carbohydrates, fats, and protein, and stay hydrated, preferring water as your main source. Take control of your energy consumption by planning meals and snacks and keeping healthy choices available. I think you are now ready to get a little more personal with your journey.

CHAPTER 3
Knowing What You Personally Need

In this chapter we explore:

- Inflammation, the silent killer
- The glycemic index eating plan
- The blood-type eating plan

INFLAMMATION, the Silent Killer

will tell you that from a health and wellness perspective, an overwhelming majority of health problems result from what is known as **inflammation**. It is known as the silent killer in the medical society. It is a localized physical condition in which part of the body becomes reddened, swollen, hot, and often painful, especially as a reaction to injury or infection. In layman's terms it is an unhealthy gathering of bodily hormones, chemicals, and microorganisms that causes dysfunction, pain, abnormalities, and so on. Picture your body as a neighborhood. If you look out in your neighborhood and see one person walking down the street, all is well. But if you see a group of teenagers, homeless people, drug dealers, and so on, it is a bit unsettling. Most neighborhoods start out fine, but over time, gangs, burglars, criminals, and the like begin to take over. This is inflammation. In your body there are defense mechanisms that are armed to take care of invaders to the body. The problem begins when your body is in a constant fight. When the body is at war with itself, it sets off a constant alarm, causing overwhelming health concerns—diabetes, high blood pressure, obesity (your neighborhood lowlifes). When the police force in your neighborhood gets overrun with crime, even they begin to tire, and the neighborhood deteriorates.

Causes of Inflammation: Inflammation can be triggered by a host of circumstances. Emotional and physical stress, infections, digestive issues, allergies, hormones just to name a few. This is why regular doctor visits are so important. For our journey here it is the nutritional trigger of inflammation that will be pursued.

Relationship Perspective: These are people everybody hates because they know these people are the opposite of everything positive in life. They break the law constantly, live a very unhealthy life, and always seem to be where you are. They don't live with you, but your life, no matter how great, is negatively affected by their presence. The only way to avoid them is to stay away from them, unfriend them, or just cut them out of your life. Most of the time it may seem they are not affecting you because they have always been part of the gang, but you've ignored them hoping you could just outlive their influence.

Insulin: Chemically, when you eat anything, but mainly carbohydrates, it must be broken down into the simplest form of glucose in order for the body to use the energy from the substance. As mentioned earlier, the more basic (simple) the substance the quicker the body will uptake the glucose. The more complex, the longer it will take to breakdown. This will cause a rise in your blood glucose level. Your pancreas detects rising blood glucose and responds by secreting insulin. Insulin is a hormone that regulates the metabolism of carbohydrates and fats by promoting the absorption of glucose, a simple sugar that is an important energy source in living organisms, from the blood to skeletal muscles and fat tissue and by causing fat to be stored rather than used for energy. When you consume food, this hormone is the usher that allows glucose to enter your cells to power your bodily processes. Insulin becomes a problem when it cannot be used for that purpose due to certain metabolic abnormalities within your internal systems. The term for this type of abnormality is "insulin resistance," which is a condition in which the body's cells become resistant to the effects of insulin. That is, the normal response to a given amount of insulin is reduced. As a result, higher levels of insulin are needed in order for insulin to have its proper effects. So the pancreas compensates by trying to produce more insulin. This resistance occurs in response to the body's own insulin or when insulin is administered by injection. With insulin resistance, the pancreas produces more and more insulin until it can no longer produce sufficient insulin for the body's demands, and then blood sugar rises. It should also be noted that insulin is a fat-storage hormone, which makes it a risk factor for development of diabetes and heart disease.

Relationship Perspective: This is the inflammation friend you're letting stay with you for a little while because he or she has nowhere else to go. This person has now over-stayed his or her welcome. Your house is a mess. You have caught that virus he or she had. You are now eating some of the unhealthy food this person eats. Doctor visits are piling up. Your only hope is tough love. Put the person out and press restart on your health.

Let's take a five-minute science break. Consuming foods that contain high amounts of fructose—even if it's a natural product—is, to put it bluntly, the fastest way to trash your health. GreenMedInfo.com has collated a number of scientific studies that have linked fructose to about thirty different specific diseases and health problems. Adding insult to injury, high-fructose corn syrup is most often made from genetically engineered corn, which is fraught with its own well-documented side effects and health concerns, from an increased risk of developing food allergies to the risk of increased infertility in future generations and possibly cancer, according to a recent lifetime feeding study.

The Glycemic Index Eating Plan

In chapter two I stated that it is not the intent of this book to advocate any specific diet as the supreme law of the land. However, there are two concepts based on scientific biochemistry that I would like to share that in my mind are not considered diets. The difference between these two concepts and a diet is that there are no hard-and-fast rules on what to eat or what not to eat. You are given scientific data, and you decide how you want to apply the data to your nutrition. Relationship-wise, it is the equivalent of an internet dating sight or speed dating system. It shows you potential partners, and you decide what you want to take a chance on. They are not rigorous regimes that must be followed to the letter but basic qualities of nutrition that allow you to make informed decisions. A buffet, if you will. So log on and begin browsing.

The glycemic index was first developed in 1981 by Dr. David Jenkins, a professor of nutrition at the University of Toronto, Canada. It was directed towards the treatment of diabetes. His research highlights the scientific fact that certain foods causes different levels of blood glucose surges. The main predictor of the surge being fiber, the more fiber a food has the slower the effect of blood glucose rise and the less chance of inflammation. Dr. Jenkins' research also suggests that the type of carbohydrate, the cooking process, and the presence of fat and dietary fiber all affect a food's glycemic index. In a person's diet, it is the glycemic index of mixed meals, referred to as the glycemic load of a meal, rather than the individual foods, that counts.

Further information is outlined in the book, "The New Glucose Revolution", by Jennie Brand-Miller, PhD, et. al. I would highly recommend this authoritative guide to the glycemic index.

My experience with this eating plan has been very positive. Being very active my whole life I never had weight-related issues until I reached the tender age of 50. I began to experience bouts of intense pain in my hip and knee brought on by prolonged standing and intense physical activity. After several doctor visits, self- medicating ventures and exercise changes I was given the ultimate diagnosis that no lifetime legend in his own mind, indestructible superhero wants to hear. "You have to lose weight!!!." At what I thought was a very muscular 205lbs was too much weight for my 50-year-old joints. Try convincing my 25-year-old mind. I was introduced to this eating plan by a coworker who I witnessed lose 30 pounds in a very short amount of time. I slowly integrated this process into my everyday eating plan and have maintained a highly manageable 185lbs for 5 years. Hip and knee pain have decreased by at least 80% in my 50 plus mind-still there but hardly noticeable. I might add that this was the only change I integrated.

Now since this is my personal infomercial, I have to end with, "results are not typical." Bio-individuality is always the common denominator when it comes to most things in life. So I will not even put a guarantee on any amount of success. So many other factors are at play that could vary results. Following is a glycemic index food list:

- LOW glycemic foods: less than 55
- MEDIUM glycemic foods: 55–70
- HIGH glycemic foods: 70 or higher

Food	GI	Serving Size (g)	GL
CANDY/SWEETS			
Honey	87	2 Tbs	17.9
Jelly Beans	78	1 oz	22
Snickers Bar	68	60g (1/2 bar)	23
Table Sugar	68	2 Tbs	7
Strawberry Jam	51	2 Tbs	10.1
Peanut M&Ms	33	30g (1 oz)	5.6
Dove Dark Chocolate Bar	23	37g (1 oz)	4.4

Food	GI	Serving Size (g)	GL
BAKED GOODS & CEREAL			
Corn Bread	110	60g (1 piece)	30.8
French Bread	95	64g (1 slice)	29.5
Corn Flakes	92	28g (1 cup)	21.1
Corn Chex	83	30g (1 cup)	20.8
Rice Krispies	82	33g (1.25 cup)	23
Corn Pops	80	31g (1 cup)	22.4
Donut (lrg. Glazed)	76	75g (1 donut)	24.3
Waffle (homemade)	76	75g (1 waffle)	18.7
Grape Nuts	75	58g (1/2 cup)	31.5
Bran Flakes	74	29g (3/4 cup)	13.3
Graham Cracker	74	14g (2 sqrs)	8.1
Cheerios	74	30g (1 cup)	13.3
Kaiser Roll	73	57g (1 roll)	21.2
Bagel	72	89g (1/4 in)	33
Corn Tortilla	70	24g (1 tortilla)	7.7
Melba Toast	70	12g (4 rounds)	5.6
Wheat Bread	70	28g (1 slice)	7.7
White Bread	70	25g (1 slice)	8.4
Kellogg's Special K	69	31g (1 cup)	14.5
Taco Shell	68	13g (1 med)	4.8
Angel Food cake	67	28g (1 slice)	10.7
Croissant, Butter	67	57g (1 med)	17.5
Muselix	66	55g (2/3 cup)	23.8
Oatmeal, Instant	65	234g (1 cup)	13.7
Rye Bread, 100% whole	65	32g (1 slice)	8.5
Rye Krisp Crackers	65	25g (1 wafer)	11.1
Raisin Bran	61	61g (1 cup)	24.4
Bran Muffin	60	113g (1 med)	30
Blueberry Muffin	59	113g (1 med)	30
Oatmeal	58	117g (1/2 cup)	64
Whole Wheat Pita	57	64g (1 pita)	17
Oatmeal Cookie	55	18g (1 large)	6
Popcorn	55	8g (1 cup)	2.8

Food	GI	Serving Size (g)	GL
BAKED GOODS & CEREAL			
Pound cake, Sara Lee	54	30g (1 piece)	8.1
Vanilla Cake and Vanilla frosting	42	64g (1 slice)	16
Pumpernickel Bread	41	26g (1 slice)	4.5
Chocolate cake w/chocolate frosting	38	64g (1 slice)	12.5

Food	GI	Serving Size (g)	GL
BEVERAGES			
Gatorade Powder	78	16g (.75 scoop)	11.7
Cranberry Juice Cocktail	68	253g (1 cup)	24.5
Cola, Carbonated	63	370g (12oz can)	25.2
Orange Juice	57	249g (1 cup)	14.25
Hot Chocolate Mix	51	28g (1 packet)	11.7
Grapefruit Juice, sweetened	48	250g (1 cup)	13.4
Pineapple juice	46	250g (1 cup)	14.37
Soy Milk	44	245g (1 cup)	4
Apple Juice	41	248g (1 cup)	11.9
Tomato Juice	38	243g (1 cup)	3.4

Food	GI	Serving Size (g)	GL
LEGUMES			
Baked Beans	48	253g (1 cup)	18.2
Pinto Beans	39	171g (1 cup)	11.7
Lima Beans	31	241g (1 cup)	7.4
Chickpeas, Boiled	31	240g (1 cup)	13.3
Lentils	29	198g (1 cup)	7
Kidney Beans	27	256g (1 cup)	7
Soy Beans	20	172g (1 cup)	1.4
Peanuts	13	146g (1 cup)	1.6

Food	GI	Serving Size (g)	GL
VEGETABLES			
Potato	104	213g (1 med)	36.4
Parsnip	97	78g (1/2 cup)	11.6
Carrot, Raw	92	15g (1 large)	1

Food	GI	Serving Size (g)	GL
Beets, canned	64	246g (1/2 cup)	9.6
Corn, yellow	55	166g (1/2 cup)	61.5
Sweet Potato	54	133g (1 cup)	12.4
Yam	51	136g (1 cup)	16.8
Peas, frozen	48	72g (1/2 cup)	3.4
Tomato	38	123g (1 med)	1.5
Broccoli, cooked	0	78g (1/2 cup)	0
Cabbage, cooked	0	75g (1/2 cup)	0
Celery, raw	0	62g (1 stalk)	0
Cauliflower	0	100g (1 cup)	0
Green Beans	0	135g (1 cup)	0
Mushrooms	0	70g (1 cup)	0
Spinach	0	30g (1 cup)	0

Food	GI	Serving Size (g)	GL
FRUIT			
Watermelon	72	152g (1 cup)	7.2
Pineapple, raw	66	155g (1 cup)	11.9
Cantaloupe	65	177g (1 cup)	7.8
Apricot, canned in light syrup	64	253g (1 cup)	24.3
Raisins	64	43g (small box)	20.5
Papaya	60	140g (1 cup)	6.6
Peaches, canned, heavy syrup	58	262g (1 cup)	28.4
Kiwi, w/skin	58	76g (1 fruit)	5.2
Fruit Cocktail, drained	55	214g (1 cup)	19.8
Peaches, canned, light syrup	52	251g (1 cup)	17.7
Banana	51	118g (1 cup)	12.2
Mango	51	165g (1 cup)	12.8
Orange	48	140g (1 fruit)	7.2
Pears, canned in pear juice	44	248g (1 cup)	12.3
Grapes	43	92g (1 cup)	6.5
Strawberries	40	152g (1 cup)	3.6
Apples, w/skin	39	138g (1 med)	6.2
Pears	33	166g (1 med)	6.9
Apricot, dried	32	130g (1 cup)	23
Prunes	29	132g (1 cup)	34.2

Peach	28	98g (1 med)	2.2
Grapefruit	25	123g (1/2 fruit)	2.8
Plum	24	66g (1 fruit)	1.7
Sweet Cheeries, raw	22	117g (1 cup)	3.7

Food	GI	Serving Size (g)	GL
NUTS			
Cashews	22		
Almonds	0		
Hazelnuts	0		
Macedamia	0		
Pecans	0		
Walnuts	0		

Food	GI	Serving Size (g)	GL
FRUIT			
Ice Cream (lower fat)	47	76g (1/2 cup)	9.2
Pudding	44	100g (1/2 cup)	8.4
Milk, Whole	40	244g (1 cup)	4.4
Ice Cream	38	72g (1/2 cup)	6
Yogurt, plain	36	245g (1 cup)	6.1

Food	GI	Serving Size (g)	GL
MEAT			
Beef	0		
Chicken	0		
Eggs	0		
Fish	0		
Lamb	0		
Pork	0		
Veal	0		
Deer-Venison	0		
Elk	0		
Buffalo	0		
Rabbit	0		
Duck	0		

Ostrich	0
Shellfish	0
Lobster	0

Follow these tips for Fat-Busting Meals:

- Avoid grains, including corn.
- Avoid potatoes and other white foods, such as white rice, sugar, and salt.
- Try making protein the focus of each meal. It kicks your metabolism into higher gear. All meats, fish, and poultry are the real "guilt-free" foods. The protein will help you handle insulin better, build muscle, and repair tissue— all essential for staying lean and preventing diabetes.
- Snack on nuts and seeds. They are a good source of protein and have omega-3s.
- Avoid processed foods, trans fats, caffeine, and high-fructose corn syrup. All increase insulin resistance.
- Choose vegetables that are low glycemic.
- Choose fruits such as berries and fruits you can eat with the skin on.
- Eat a high-protein breakfast every morning. It will stabilize your blood sugar and get you off to a good start.

I don't consider the glycemic index principle a diet. It gives you scientifically based information on the real properties of food items and leaves it up to the individual to choose. It is with this concept that I lost twenty pounds relatively fast. I will not tell you how fast because that could be unique to me. That might not fit into your puzzle. Learn more about the glycemic index at (http://nutritiondata.self.com/topics/glycemic-index)

The Blood Type Eating Plan

We've all heard the term that blood is thicker than water. Hopefully we all know that means if you are related to someone by blood you have a closer bond with them than you would to someone who is not. Our blood does a lot of wonderful things for us such as:

- Supply of oxygen to tissues
- Supply of nutrients such as glucose, amino acids, and fatty acids

- Removal of waste such as carbon dioxide, urea, and lactic acid
- Immunological functions, including circulation of white blood cells, and detection of foreign material by antibodies
- Coagulation, the response to a broken blood vessel, the conversion of blood from a liquid to a semi-solid gel to stop bleeding
- Messenger functions, including the transport of hormones and the signaling of tissue damage
- Regulation of body pH
- Regulation of core body temperature

You can see by this list that we need to have a good relationship with our blood. Once again, I believe this to be a relationship of necessity and not just casual friendship. Just as two people may not be compatible in a relationship, your blood has a unique relationship with you. As far as nutrition is concerned the most important part of our blood are antigens. An antigen is any substance that causes an immune system to produce antibodies against it. An antibody is a protein used by the body to neutralize harmful substances in our bodies. From a relationship perspective these are our defense mechanisms that keep us feeling safe and secure. Some people have a need to be social so they will gravitate to social situations. Others need solitude so they will choose to be alone for security. These reactions are the antigens and antibodies of our wellbeing. According to *Eat Right 4 Your Type, by Dr. Peter J. D'Adamo and Catherine Whitney*, different blood types have different antigens that react uniquely to the environment they are in. Their research contends that these differences in blood type antigens in that unique environment causes a varied response to metabolism and nutrition. They conclude that choosing the foods for your blood type will allow you to lose weight, reduce inflammation, increase energy, and lead a longer, healthier life. I have personally experimented with this unique plan of selective food choices for my blood type with very positive results. My weight has been stabilized, my energy level has been elevated and my seasonal allergies have been almost become nonexistent just to name a few positives. As with all things on this journey the concept of bio-individuality is the overarching theme. Because of the host of biological, chemical and genetic influences with all people, there is no bottom line right or wrong choice until it is tested. The only suggestion I would assign to this plan is to stay as natural as possible with any choice and the body will respond naturally sending either positive or negative signals. I recommend you going to http://www.dadamo.com or reading

Dr. D'Adamos' book to obtain further information on food lists and other suggestions for each blood type.

As stated earlier, these are not hard-and-fast rules that restrict any food group, but they give you information to make informed decisions about your nutrition relationship. These choices may work for you or they may not be for you. I've personally had success with both but the laws of bio-individuality can be applied to a number of things in health and wellness as we have learned.

Summary: Life is about choices. Relationships are about choices. The "die" in the word "diet" means most if not all diets end up in failure because of the lack of sustainability. They are so restricting that people view them as a prison sentence, and they spend most of their time waiting for parole. This in and of itself is unhealthy. Recognizing and managing inflammation puts you in the driver's seat of controlling your daily health, which in turn improves your quality of life substantially. The glycemic index and blood-type eating plans are all about choice and freedom. You are given the keys to the car. Just follow the traffic laws. You can go five miles over or under without getting a ticket.

Relationship Perspective: It is like speed dating. You have limited contact with no commitment, but you still have a good time. But in every endeavor, there are temptations and roadblocks that you must deal with. Half the battle is just knowing your enemy and their weaknesses. There are two major enemies in this warfare. First the subtle spy within our own camp. Thinking we are invincible and can make it without a plan. This fades away quickly with mounting doctor visits from constant weekend warrior relationship events. Second is the temptations that are placed in our path to entice us to just try a little sip of this or a taste of that before we have enough experience in the game. Think before you act.

CHAPTER 4

Mind And Body Connection/Cravings

In this chapter we explore:

- The possible origins of your food cravings
- Strategies to deal with food cravings
- Nutritional Crowd Control

opefully, I've stated the obvious to most people: that we need food and water to survive. Oftentimes we tend to oversimplify things, causing us some degree of problems in our existence. It should help to understand why we need these sources and how they serve us.

Now, our bodies internally know what they need. As stated earlier, they are highly adaptable to many changing environments, mental and emotional states, physical adjustments, and a host of other changes we are subject to. The more we connect with this internal functioning, the better we are able to serve the body to its standards. And when it is served correctly, it will respond with better internal regulation, metabolic functioning, hormonal balance, immune functioning, weight management, and mental performance, among many other positive quality-of-life issues. The problem comes when one's mind becomes sabotaged with constant advertisements of the almighty pleasure principle, so to speak. And where the mind goes, the body will follow.

Let's face it: we live in a world full of visions of what perfect is for everybody. So many people and organizations would be left jobless or out of business if they couldn't appeal to the pursuit of perfection. If we buy into the society model of perfection, we tend to develop what is considered a craving, which is a strong desire for something. As mentioned earlier, we see the perfect body, the successful career, the popular personality, and somehow convince ourselves that this is what will make us happy. Very seldom do we stop and consider what might lie beneath. Nutritionally, for that space in time when we're presented with an advertisement for unhealthy choices, we depart from our basic-need instinct and enter into our fantasy castle, if you will, and suppress what is needed. Here is the bottom line. If we know something is bad for us or not in our best interests and we still have to have it, there is a mind-body disconnect and we force our bodies to give us signals as to the consequences of our actions. No one is immune. As health-conscious as I am, if you put a container of peppermint patties in front of me and leave, you might want know how many were in the container. My defense against this addiction is not having it in my home. So in order for me to have it, it must find me. That's a neat trick if you can pull it off. One final thing before we explore how to deal with cravings. A common response from some of us when confronted with the "Why do we eat something that is bad for us?" line is "Life is too short for me not to be happy." Well, if your happiness is attached to food, there might be a deeper issue.

Many people view cravings as weaknesses, but really they are important messages meant to assist us in maintaining balance. When we experience a craving, my Integrative Nutrition® training teaches deconstruction. Ask yourself, what does my body want and why? Here are some of the things I have learned.

1. Everything in our lives that we have to deal with requires energy for us to be healthy and successful. Once we recognize this it will be easier for us to look at these energy sources as food that either sustains us or drains us. Therefore, any relationship, job, endeavor or practice needs to be evaluated and managed to bring us into balance with what our true purpose is. If it is a constant energy drain, adjust or make plans to eliminate it.

2. Our bodies are to a large degree made up of water and craves water for normal function and recovery. Staying hydrated could be the answer to certain cravings. Problems arise when our taste buds take over and we listen to those signals over our natural need.

3. As explained earlier, our systems know what it needs and will constantly send us signals if we don't give it what it needs. Real food, unprocessed carbs, good fats and protein, has very few substitutes. Relationships often fail when someone goes outside of the relationship because they crave something that their partner is not giving them. Normally there is a period of craving prior to the event, ie. a lack of affection, waning interests, financial insecurity or a host of other necessary relationship food.

4. Everyone is familiar with the emotional side of eating. We call most of it comfort food. For me it's peppermint patties which is not the worst craving. There is a certain calm and excitement in just the anticipation of tasting one. The problem with this type of craving is often portion control which will be discussed later. Too much of anything is not good for you. Or, just find a healthier version of the peppermint patty. You can also talk to any woman who has been pregnant and ask what her craving was.

5. Holidays are very important cultural food staples. Christmas means several varieties of cookies, fruit cake and egg nog. Easter means chocolate covered eggs. Thanksgiving means varieties of pies, turkey and assorted sweets. The list is quite extensive, not to mention the religious influences. Just like any other relationship, knowing your partner and communication can assist with this type of craving.

Just like anything else in life that gives recommendations for problems, trial and error for your particular situation is the standard. Sometimes just being aware of certain principles causes positive thoughts, which transfer to the body and, in turn, into behavior.

I have never been a fan of sequels. I always believe you can't improve on an original. This is not to say that there is never room for improvement. It depends on what you are trying to improve upon. In this day and time, we are inundated with constant improvement. Technology turnaround is so fast you need to change devices increasingly faster. We have experienced a food turnaround that has resulted in our not being able to recognize the food we grew up with. It has been stripped of the natural necessities we need to achieve true health and wellness.

We are living creatures, and our bodies grow and perform better ingesting things that are alive or have lived. Now, all you animal rights or other groups, please bear with me. There are just certain things only your mother or grandmother can prepare that satisfy you. They use some of the same ingredients but in different quantities or preparation methods. From a religious standpoint, I believe God—or, if you don't believe in God, the earth as it evolved—provides everything we need to be healthy and well. You can find things sweet, sour, salty, bitter, and with various textures and other experiences growing from the earth. Contrary to popular belief, all animals are edible and provide protein that serves the human body. I will spare you the scriptures because I don't want to lose those who will actually stop and look it up. Now, we all know that some people have an aversion or allergies to certain foods, and that is real.

Obviously those people need to follow certain guidelines from their physicians. The bottom line is that if you give your body what it basically needs and stick with the original recipe it was designed to ingest, it will respond by giving you the best return on your investment.

Nutritional Crowd Control

To use an old TV legendary saying, "Space, the final frontier". We often hear how one of humans' major concerns is overcrowding. This single phenomenon could cause a ripple effect in the quality of life to whoever is affected. We see it everywhere. If you get on an elevator there is a weight or people limit. In all gathering places the fire marshal will be summoned if the number of people exceed the limit. A percentage of people suffer from claustrophobia which is the extreme or irrational fear of confined places. And finally it has made it into our nutritional systems. "Can I supersize that for you?", "For just 50 cents more you can get an extra burger and small fry" or whatever the large Starbucks coffee is called now.

Relationship Perspective: It is no secret that a majority of us need our space. We are sometimes called anti-social if we don't come and join the crowd for drinks or to just hang out. I believe if you are in constant need of social interaction you may need to strive for a balance in your relationships. There is a possibility of a dependency issue that could arise. But I'm not a psychiatrist nor psychologist so take it with a grain of sodium, but not too much. On the other hand our journey is all about bio-individuality. So try to spend some time being comfortable with you and I believe that is the start of you finding that balance. Now let's take a look at some of the factors that can affect our nutritional quality balance.

Portion size: Portion size plays a role in how much we eat. When people select their own portions, the size of the serving bowl may affect the amount consumed. We tend to respond visually to the amount of food on a plate or the size of a serving utensil and consider that "normal" rather than paying attention to internal feelings of satiation. The dramatic increase in portion sizes eaten both at home and at restaurants may be a major contributing factor to excess energy intake and weight gain.

Environmental and Social Factors: We tend to eat more in cold weather and less in hot weather. Plate size, lighting, and socializing are other factors that influence consumption.

Any change in our surroundings that inhibits our self-monitoring of consumption tends to increase the volume that we eat. Studies show that meals eaten with other people last longer and tend to increase consumption by at least one-third compared with eating alone.

Emotional Factors: Many people use food to cope with stress and negative feelings. Eating can provide a powerful distraction from loneliness, anger, boredom, anxiety, shame, sadness, and inadequacy. To combat low moods, low energy levels, and low self-esteem, people often turn to the refrigerator. When we use food and eating to cope with our emotions, binge eating or other disturbed eating patterns can develop.

Gastrointestinal Sensations As food fills your stomach and small intestine, they stretch and trigger signals to the brain. Your sense of fullness suppresses your urge to eat. Just passing a reasonable amount of food through the mouth can satisfy hunger temporarily even if the food never reaches the stomach. As we taste, salivate, chew, and swallow, the brain probably measures the passage of food, much as a water meter measures the flow of water. After a certain amount of food passes through the mouth, hunger diminishes for 20 to 40 minutes.

Neurological and Hormonal Factors: More than 50 different chemicals are thought to be involved in the regulation of feeding. We will look at two of the major hormones.

Ghrelin: Sometimes called the "hunger hormone," is produced in the stomach. Ghrelin levels rise prior to a meal and fall quickly after food is consumed. The rise in ghrelin levels appears to encouraging feeding.

Leptin: Sometimes called the "satiety hormone," is produced in fat cells. Leptin tells the central nervous system how much fat the body is storing. A rise in leptin levels appears to suppress appetite. Leptin also appears to signal pathways that enhance energy production to keep body weight in a normal range.

Unfortunately, when body weight is high, these regulators act inconsistently.

Sticking with the concept of knowledge is power, just being aware of these factors is a somewhat call to action to produce strategies to combat the negative effects of them. From a relationship perspective learn how to just say no to some social gatherings if you know they are your triggers for overeating. If by chance you are required to attend out of occupational obligations, form strategies to put in play. Life is about choices and strategies. To assist with your special planning here is a list of normal portion size equivalents:

GRAINS: 1 cup of dry cereal=4 golf balls

2 oz Bagel=1 hockey puck

½ cup cooked cereal, rice, or pasta=1 tennis ball

VEGETABLES: 1 cup of vegetables=1 baseball or a rubiks cube

FRUITS: 1 medium fruit (equivalent of 1 cup of fruit)=1 baseball

FLUIDS: 1 tsp vegetable oil=1 die (11/16)

1 tbsp salad dressing= 1 jacks ball

MEAT: 3 oz cooked meat=1 deck of playing cards

CHESSE: 11/2 oz of hard cheese=6 dice

1/3 cup of shredded cheese=1 billiard or racquet ball

Summary: The toughest battles are those that we wage against ourselves. The disconnect from our natural instinct to be healthy comes with signals like idiot lights on a car dashboard. The non-mechanic will oftentimes wait to see if the light will go off on its own in an attempt to save money on a visit. Relationship wise, it's "Something doesn't seem right feeling with this person, but let's give it one more week and see where this goes because I really want this to work." Take the car in and have the mechanic tell you what is wrong. Tell the person, "We need some time apart so I can collect myself" and see what he or she says. Our final enemy is not so subtle. He or she knows our weakness and attacks it overtly, head on.

CHAPTER 5

The Nutritional Dating Scene

In this chapter we explore:

- The several forms of sugar
- How the body processes sugar vs. glucose
- Strategies for food shopping and dining out
- Food label reading

Love at First Sight—So It Seems: As you seek out a partner in any relationship, it is always advisable to first know what you are looking for, what you are not looking for, and, last but certainly not least, what is good for you. Chapter 1 should have covered a vast amount of information to help you with these important decisions. It is at this point that we must distinguish between a few identities of relationship warfare.

Hunger: A feeling of discomfort or weakness caused by lack of food, coupled with the desire to eat. It is the physical desire for food. Nutritionally speaking it is our stomach churning or growling as a signal that our energy stores have been depleted and more is needed. Obviously this is a constant life survival situation that must be balanced appropriately. No science required here. The relationship equivalent of this would be the person that constantly needs to be in a relationship and hasn't been in one in a while. They will see other couples enjoying each other and become physically and mentally stressed out.

Appetite: A natural desire to satisfy a bodily need, especially for food. It is a psychological desire for food. It arouses our senses at the smell, sight or maybe even the sound of something cooking. Now we all know much too well the power of the mind and how it can lead to action. The relationship equivalent of this is the ever present attraction to a mate, whether they are attainable or not. The curves, look or sent of a woman. The muscles, strength or attire of a man. Some have healthy appetites while others are a little more satisfied with little.

Satiety: To fill or supply beyond capacity or desire, often arousing weariness. Nutritionally speaking it is the point at which our hunger is satisfied. As we all know too well there is no shut-off valve to the stomach. That extra intake must go somewhere so the body will either store it as fat or use it for energy-Your choice. The obvious relationship connection here is very extensive. Too many mates can drain energy, stress the mind, physically attack immune systems, just to name a few.

Now in a perfect world, hunger and appetite were meant to work together to bring the body into nutritional balance. It is at this point you will meet a pair of siblings in the nutrition relationship world that you must be aware of. One is a very manipulative entity—or nutritional terrorist, if you will—that is ever present. It presents itself in a very high-maintenance appearance, has the ability to temporarily satisfy all your immediate hunger desires—not needs—takes the form of everything in your wildest fantasies, and occupies a major portion of your heart and soul if you let it. The other, even though from the same family, represents itself very modestly, gives you what you need for the moment, and provides you with pleasant conversation and a lasting, true friendship—but not an intimate relationship. But if you hang around with it too much, it has the potential to take on the characteristics of its related family member. So it is something of a balancing act not to hang out with either one too often. The danger is in the collateral damage that could plague your life...uh, relationship health. Sound intriguing? It is...

Sugar

I did not put this substance in the previous chapter because that chapter was about needs. This chapter is about managing the battle of wants and needs. There are two types of sugars in American diets: naturally occurring sugars and added sugars. The other type of sugar, glucose, is manufactured by the body after consumption of macronutrients, carbohydrates, fats, and protein and then used by cells for energy. To understand the impact of sugar on your system, you must understand how the body breaks down these sugars.

First, the natural: Naturally occurring sugars are found *naturally* in foods such as fruit (fructose) and milk (lactose). This is the good sibling. The natural part is the good of this relationship. Because it is natural, there are other good metabolites such as fiber, vitamins, and minerals combined in most of these sugars—hence the good conversation and friendship. Because they are sugars, you still need to watch how much time you give these relationships. You might recognize these examples as being the same as simple carbohydrates. Let's give them a hand as they come back onstage:

- Fruit
- Milk
- Milk products

I will expand the discussion of these sugars further to show how they are used—metabolized—by the body.

Now, the added: Added sugars include *any* sugars or caloric sweeteners that are *added* to foods or beverages during processing or preparation (such as putting sugar in your coffee or adding sugar to your cereal). Added sugars (or added sweeteners) can include natural sugars such as white sugar, brown sugar, and honey, as well as other caloric sweeteners that are chemically manufactured (such as high-fructose corn syrup). Let's give them a hand as they come back onstage. Feel free to boo if you like. They know how bad they are:

- Candy
- Table sugar
- Syrups
- Soft drinks
- Pastries

Relationship Perspective: Sugars are similar to your bad-fat friends in that their appearance is breathtaking. They have that silver tongue and even know how to make your relatives feel good about them. Everybody likes the sweet person. In reality they are spies from the enemy. Terrorists, if you will. Once they have befriended you and skillfully painted themselves onto your canvas, they begin to eat away at you quietly. And before you know it, things begin to fall apart. If these tactics are not dealt with as soon as possible, your credit is wrecked, self-esteem shot, immune system compromised, and identity in question. This enemy is by far the most dangerous adversary in relationship history—the black plague of the modern relationship story. Let's go to science class for a few minutes.

Scientists using newer functional magnetic resonance imaging (fMRI) tests have now shown that fructose, a sugar found in most processed foods (typically in the form of high-fructose corn syrup), can in fact trigger changes in your brain that may lead to overeating and weight gain.

The researchers discovered that when you drink a beverage containing fructose, your brain does not register the feeling of being satiated, as it does when you consume simple glucose.

How Your Body Metabolizes Fructose Versus Glucose

Part of what makes fructose so unhealthy is that it is *metabolized by your liver to fat* far more rapidly than any other sugar. The entire burden of metabolizing fructose falls on your liver, and it promotes visceral fat. This is the type of fat that collects around your organs and in your abdominal region and is associated with a greater risk of heart disease.

Without getting into the complex biochemistry of carbohydrate metabolism, it is important to understand how your body processes fructose versus glucose. Dr. Robert Lustig, professor of pediatrics in the Division of Endocrinology at the University of California, has been a pioneer in decoding sugar metabolism. His work has highlighted some major differences in how different sugars are broken down and used. Here's a summary of the main points:

- After you've eaten fructose, 100 percent of the metabolic burden rests on your liver. With glucose, your liver has to break down only 20 percent. The metabolism of fructose by your liver creates a long list of waste products and toxins, including a large amount of uric acid, which drives up blood pressure and causes gout.
- Gout is a type of arthritis characterized by painful, stiff, and inflamed joints. The stiffness and swelling are a result of excess uric acid forming crystals in

your joints, and the pain associated with this disease is caused by your body's inflammatory response to the crystals.

- Every cell in your body, including your brain, utilizes glucose. Therefore, much of it is "burned up" immediately after you consume it. By contrast, fructose is turned into free fatty acids (FFAs), VLDL (the damaging form of cholesterol), and triglycerides, which get stored as fat.
- The fatty acids created during fructose metabolism accumulate as fat droplets in your liver and skeletal muscle tissues, causing insulin resistance and nonalcoholic fatty liver disease (NAFLD). Insulin resistance progresses to metabolic syndrome and type 2 diabetes.
- When you eat 120 calories of glucose, less than 1 calorie is stored as fat. Eating 120 calories of fructose results in 40 calories being stored as fat.
- Glucose suppresses your hunger hormone ghrelin and stimulates leptin, which suppresses your appetite. Fructose has no effect on ghrelin and interferes with your brain's communication with leptin, resulting in overeating.

Now, for those of you who must have the sweet nectar on occasion, there are natural and artificial sweeteners out there. I will not go into detail because research is still being done on the effects of most. I will leave you with information to do your own research.

OK. If that is not enough to scare you straight, then experience will have to be your best teacher. I hope this will not be the case for you.

The Pursuit of Happiness: If it is not painfully obvious at this point, having a positive self-relationship is the best start to finding the right partner. Once you have conquered that Mount Everest, you will have a clearer perspective on what lies below. It would be great if the story could end there and we all live happily ever after. The mantra goes like this: "I'm happy all by myself." "I don't need a man or woman to make me happy." Or "I'm through with people." We all know that life does not work like that. You have to go to work, you have to leave the house, you have to talk to or have some type of human interaction or relationship at some level, and it will have some impact on your life and/or health. It's all a matter of how you manage the relationship.

Now, a main issue with finding a relationship is where to look. I'm going to walk softly here because I don't think anyone has the statistics on the ultimate, guaranteed, never-miss, compatibility-sure, it-will-last-forever hookup place. And even if there were such a statistic, somebody would dive in and it would not work for that person. People have met in all places and situations. Some have worked out, and others have failed. It's all about relationship management. But in the nutrition love affair, where you meet matters a great deal. Let's look at a few of the nutritional considerations and hot spots out there.

THE FINANCIAL COST OF A RELATIONSHIP: Finance has been the Achilles heel of many relationships. Disagreement over how much, where to or when to spend are common roadblocks to the casual and legal unions.

EATING OUT: According to thesimpledollar.com, the average American eats out between four and **five times** a week at an average cost of **$12.75** per meal. It is calculated that the average American would save **$36.75 per person** per week. For most, relaxation, atmosphere, occasion, status or many other reasons are worth the investment for eating out. Whether this is a good or bad meeting place depends on who is at that location. Most fast-food restaurants are nothing more than controlled nightclubs filled with your everyday simple sugars, processed carbohydrates, and fried or baked unhealthy fats. Obviously they are dressed to impress, adorned with elegant aromas and sparkling jewelry. They are difficult to resist and should only be visited sparingly if at all. Depending on your willpower and life station, they can be disastrous to your relationship status and health. Your more upscale restaurants are a safer bet, and you will find more of the people who are compatible with your profile and health. You will see more sophisticated people such as entrees, soups of the day, vegetables, and, yes, water. The problem with any of these hookup places is fear of the unknown. How was the food prepared? Am I allergic to any of the ingredients? Did the cooks wash their hands? Are the ingredients fresh? There are many more that can be added to this list. Last, but certainly not least, is the drain on one of your most precious resources/finances. When it comes to finances, these people are high-maintenance relationships. Consider this: You need gas money, clothes, jewelry, the possibility of getting a ticket, traffic, parking, and, last but not least, the price of the food. This is not a cheap or reasonable date most of the time. He/she may make you feel good and they probably look good on your resume of places you have eaten and you may even enjoy the socialization, but the feeling is temporary and you have less money for other things. Bottom line: Unless you have an endless supply of cash flow or all those other factors outweigh your financial need, try to limit the number of visits if you can. Don't get me wrong, I love the occasional dining out experience for special events or just to treat myself at some point, but I try not to make a long-term commitment to this partner.

EATING AT HOME: Obviously, this is the most successful meeting place of all. It is safe, affordable, without traffic or parking issues, and very reasonable to your budget. You don't have to dress up, the bathrooms should be well maintained (or at least you have some control of that), and the positive list goes on and on. The only negative on this list is whom you allow into the establishment. You see, you control the menu, how the food is prepared, the atmosphere, the entertainment, and many other aspects of the experience. At any time it can be a five-star restaurant, a small café on the corner, a healthy fast-food experience, a snack bar—the possibilities are endless. Now, to make this meeting place the best it can be, some of us may have to do an overhaul to the establishment. Up to this point, the place may have allowed some pretty shady characters to hang out in and around the establishment. With a little education and dedication, you can change your personal relationship meeting place into a fine, delicious, intimate dining experience. Stay tuned. If I can go so far as to make a bold suggestion to make this experience even more pleasurable, take pride in this relationship. Make preparing your own food somewhat of an intimate experience. Nutritional foreplay if you will. It is like the boy or girl next door that you grew up with. You know everything about them and what to expect from them. The relationship has always been one of trust and true friendship. They have always been there for you. They have what you need. For a little perspective I will give you my weekly dinner grocery bill:

Salad

ITEM	PRICE/AMOUNT	# OF SERV.	TOTAL
Baby Spinach	$4.77 container	10	0.48
Cucumber	0.45 1	10	0.05
Roma Tomatoes	$1.01 4	10	0.10
Broccoli Florets	$2.48 bag	10	0.25
Red Wine Vinaigrette	$1.98 bottle	16	0.12
1 Salad			**1.00**

Meal

ITEM	PRICE/AMOUNT	# OF SERV.	TOTAL
Frozen Blackeye peas	$1.48 bag	5	0.30
Frozen Chopped Spinach	$1.28 bag	5	0.26
Uncle bens Boil-in-Bag	$1.93 4 packs	8	0.24
Roasted Turkey Breast	$9.99	10	$1.00
1 Meal			**$1.80**
1 Totally Intimate Nutritional Experience			**$2.80**

Now as you have probably noticed, the numbers were rounded up or down a few cents. Serving sizes can be manipulated either way. You can substitute other items that may bring the price up or down a few notches. I don't think I have to do any more math to show you how economical and nutritious this date can be. Give the boy or girl next door a try.

SHOPPING: This is a must. Unless you have a service that does your shopping for you, you have to manage this meeting place yourself. I know you may have heard this before, but it is so true. Shop the outer perimeter of your grocery store. This is where the produce and natural foods hang out. It is a safe place to meet. The people are old school, with traditional values such as fruits, vegetables, meats, and dairy, among other safe food choices. Now, you will have to occasionally go out to the club, the inner aisles. The club does have some good people who are there just to have a good time. But you will also find all your shallow, self-centered, catch-phrase players. The music is loud. The choices are varied. But with the proper education, you can spot these simple sugars and processed carbohydrates a mile away for what they really are: candy, pastries, cereal, and bread, just to name a few. Spend very little time at the club. Those players are very persuasive and have heavy agendas. Before you know it, you will be taking one of them home. Grab your oatmeal, seasonings, and other healthy options, and run out the door.

MISCELANEOUS: This category of meeting place is that chance meeting that happens every so often and catches you off guard. When you are minding your own business and you see him or her. As mentioned earlier, the family reunion, the office party, the wedding, or any special occasion. You see that special dish or dessert, and it captivates you for the moment. Simple sugar taboo be damned! I must have it. It is OK in moderation. Go ahead and indulge. As the saying goes, "life is too short," or "stop and eat the chocolate roses along the way." The problem is taking him or her home with you and starting a torrid affair. You get the recipe so you have him or her at your leisure. It is a slippery slope—approach with caution.

STAYING IN YOUR LANE: It is a known fact and one that I have proven through experience that as we get older our nutritional needs change. Normally it is in the area of vitamins, minerals and some macro-nutrients depending on a myriad of biological and genetic factors. I will not attempt to give authoritative information on this. The only information I will impart here is to get annual physical exams, listen to your body and respond to the cues. I believe this is a bio-individuality thing. What you consumed easily at 18 years old might give you some problems at 30, 40 or 50 and beyond. From a relationship perspective it is best to stay with the food, I mean the people, as close to your era as possible. Not that 20 to 30 years difference will not work, but it usually takes a lot more effort because of different frames of reference. Obviously there are exceptions to this rule but they are normally few and far between.

Testing Your Partner / Reading Food labels: A major battle to overcome in the relationship war is the answer to the ultimate question: "Are you who you say you are?" Many relationships have been sabotaged by spies or replicas claiming to be the real thing. And they are very convincing unless you know how to uncover the wolf in sheep's clothing. It's as if someone has blindfolded you and is now feeding you something as a taste test. Let us take a quick look behind the mask and show you how to reveal the true identity of your potential partner.

Food labels: Specific federal regulations control what can and cannot appear on a food label and what must appear on it. The Food and Drug Administration (FDA) is responsible for ensuring that foods sold in the United States are safe, wholesome, and properly labeled.

Nutrition Facts Panel

1. **Serving Size:** The serving size is a standardized reference amount, but check twice to see if this is the amount you usually eat. The numbers that you will be looking at are based on this quantity.
2. **Calories per Serving:** Having the number of calories and the number of calories from fat next to each other makes it easy to see if a food is high in fat.
3. **Percent Daily Values:** These percentages are based on the values given below in the footnote for a two-thousand-calorie diet. Thus, if your caloric intake is different, you will need to adjust these values appropriately.
4. **List of Nutrients:** A list of the amounts of total fat, saturated fat, trans fat, cholesterol, sodium, total carbohydrate, dietary fiber, sugars, and protein in one serving. This information is given both in quantity (grams or milligrams per serving) and as a percentage of the daily value—a comparison standard

specifically for food labels (this standard is described in the following section). Listed next are percentages of daily values for vitamins A and C, calcium, and iron, which are the only micronutrients that must appear on all standard labels. Manufacturers may choose to include information about other nutrients, such as potassium, polyunsaturated fat, additional vitamins, or other minerals in the Nutrition Facts panel.

5. **Caloric Conversion Information:** Handy reference values help you check the math on your own calculations!

I have included a few examples of food labels to show you how these partners compete for your consumption, time, and love and/or affection. In very little time, you will become an expert at seeing food/people for what/who they really are. Some are identified, and others are left to your discretion. It is important that you pay attention to all the information to make an informed decision as to whom you spend your time or health with. There is a lot more to be said about food labeling, but this should give you a start on your journey to a healthy relationship.

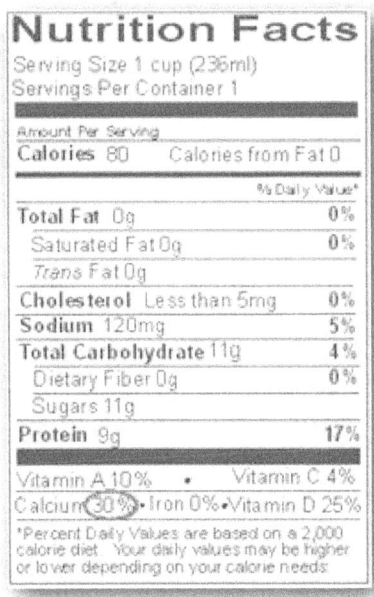
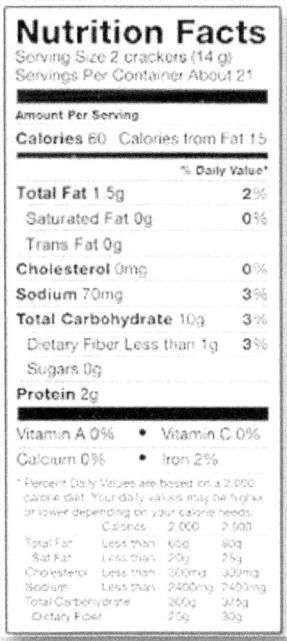

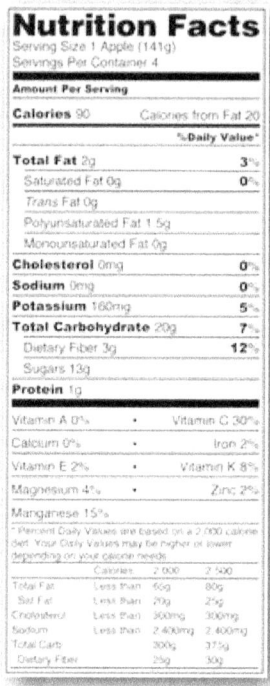

Summary: As mentioned earlier, life is about choices. Conversely, life is also about taking control. The beginning of taking control is education. Knowledge is truly power. Simply knowing something oftentimes gives people the upper hand in anything. You can either get it from a book or through life experience. They say experience is the best teaching. I believe it is best not to experience some things and benefit from the experiences of others or possibly scientific research. Nutritionally, added sugar is the most harmful substance for our health. It is also the most alluring product on the market. Relationship-wise, it is viewed as having the total package for what we want—not need. Science has proved that it has the controlling, addicting power of a narcotic. It must be avoided at all costs for us to be as well as we can. So make it your duty to be on your guard at all times—shopping, eating out, or any eating situation.

CHAPTER 6
We Need to Talk/Food Dairy

There comes a time in most relationships when one of the partners, most often the more sensitive one of the union, will utter the painful, thought-provoking and defining statement, "WE NEED TO TALK". At this point the other partner is placed in one of several states. I can't possibly name them all but surprise, relief, fear, confusion and all out stress are just a few. Normally the utterance of such a strong statement means that partner has had several ah ha moments, little bouts of reflection or experienced some unpleasant moments. Now he/she has had time to sit down, make a list, journal or maybe even produce a full written, published document on the issues at hand. They are now fed up with how the relationship is or was being managed by either partner and now is the time for a different strategy or 12 step program. The unfortunate or maybe unbelievable thing about reaching this point is that many of us spend years in unsatisfying relationships for many understandable and justifiable reasons. It is the same concept for the nutritional relationship. We know what is bad for us but it tastes so good. It is not easy to break a habit or craving that you have become accustom to even though it may not be in your best interest. People on the outside often criticize people for remaining in those relationships without trying to walk a mile in their shoes of which nobody can.

Let's go a little deeper on relationship management. There is a suggestion out there in the relationship management world that proclaims a woman needs a certain amount of touches each day to feel wanted/needed. It is contended If they do not get that level of attention, certain possible unpleasant behaviors will ensue. I will not go into detail because bio-individuality applies. Now I will not attempt to pass on exact numbers at this point because as with all things bio-individuality will play a role in this also. Having been in relationships most of my life, I'm inclined to believe this little nugget of information as I have been a frequent violator of the statute personally. Let's all come to somewhat of a consensus that this is true for most women. Oh and to be fair, most men only need a television, food, a bed and an efficient plumbing system. I have done extensive research in that field. Back to the issue at hand. Our metabolism is like a woman. It needs to be touched or somewhat attended to several times a day. A touch to the metabolism is a meal or possibly water. Now contrary to popular belief, the term meal is symbolic and not a license to eat an entrée' with potatoes, green beans and dessert at every meal. There are big meals and small meals. It could be almonds and string cheese, some beef or turkey jerky or a salad. These are considered snacks but meals none the less. Meals keep the metabolism happy and warm. And a warm metabolism can handle much more fuel and use that fuel more efficiently. Left to cool down, a cold metabolism will ultimately shut down and store any other food as fat to survive until the next scheduled fueling. I will let your mind translate that into the woman scenario.

From a nutritional perspective I recommend our intake of fuel come to that defining junction if we have been struggling in a bad nutritional relationship. Often times it may be one event (doctor visit) or a series of chronic painful health related issues that cause us to take inventory of our intake. The first step could be to get somewhat anal about our food. This is not an easy task but consider the possibility that you have been nutritionally cheated on, abused, lied to and psychologically injured. Now there are several websites and apps out there that assist with this: https://www.supertracker.usda.gov/foodtracker.aspx, http://www.bodybuilding.com/fun/nutrient.htm, and http://hnrca.tufts.edu/restaurant-meal-calculator/, just to name a few. I choose to chart this process myself because I believe in the rewards of good hard work and it doesn't help that I'm technologically lazy. Below you will find my food dairy for one day of eating. I got the information from the actual food labels on the items. Now you may not want to fill in all the categories but calories, fats, protein, carbohydrates, sugar and fiber should be the minimum from my perspective. There are more substances you can track if you would prefer. Do this for 3 days without changing anything in your eating behavior. This is your baseline and will explain a lot about how you look, feel, perform or any other health and wellness issue you wish to change. Honesty is the best policy in any relationship. Remember that you are now fed up with this current relationship. Now use the information you have learned to make informed changes incrementally and track changes according to your specific criteria; weight loss, improved blood pressure or cholesterol levels, more energy, etc. After a while you will not need the dairy as often because your relationship will become rock solid and the "just like riding a bicycle" analogy will apply.

BREAKFAST-7:00 AM AFTER WORKOUT

FOOD ITEM	SERV.	CAL	CARBS	FATS SAT	UNSAT	TRANS	PROTEIN	FIBER	SUGAR
Oatmeal	½ cup	150	27	0	2	0	5	4	1
Turkey Bacon	2 strips	80	2	0	3	0	6	0	0
Egg Whites	2	160	0	0	0	0	5	0	0
Almonds	1 Pack	100	3	1	8	0	3	2	1
Banana	1 Med	105	27	0	0	0	1.3	3.1	14.4
Blueberries	1/2cup	42	21	0	0	0	1	2	7.5
String Cheese	1 Stick	60	0	2.5	1.5	0	7	0	0
TOTALS:		697	80	3.5	14.5	0	28.3	11.1	22.9

SNACK-10:30 AM

FOOD ITEM	SERV.	CAL	CARBS	FATS SAT	UNSAT	TRANS	PROTEIN	FIBER	SUGAR
Almonds	1 Pack	100	3	1	8	0	3	2	1
TOTALS:		100	3	1	8	0	3	2	1

LUNCH-12:00 PM SALAD

FOOD ITEM	SERV.	CAL	CARBS	FATS SAT	UNSAT	TRANS	PROTEIN	FIBER	SUGAR
Salad Dress. Red Wine Vin.	2 tbls.	85	7	1	3.5	0	0	0	4
Roasted Turkey	56g	80	6	0.5	1.5	0	5	0	2
Spinach /raw	3 cups	20	3	0	0	0	2	2	0
Broccoli /raw	1 Cup	25	4	0	0	0	3	3	1

Food Item	Serv.	CAL	CARBS	SAT	UNSAT	TRANS	PROTEIN	FIBER	SUGAR
Cucumber	1/4	30	5	0	0	0	0.5	2	0
Tomato	1/2 Md.	11	2.4	0.1	0.3	0	1.0	1.5	3.0
Sun Chips	1 oz	140	18	1	4.5	0	2	3	2
String Cheese	1 Stick	60	0	2.5	1.5	0	7	0	0
TOTALS:		**551**	**45.4**	**5.1**	**11.3**	**0**	**20.5**	**9.5**	**12**

SNACK-2:30 – 3:00 PM
FATS

FOOD ITEM	SERV.	CAL	CARBS	SAT	UNSAT	TRANS	PROTEIN	FIBER	SUGAR
Carrots	3 oz bag	35	8	0	0	0	1	2	5
Apple	1 med	72	19.1	0	0.1	0	0.4	3.3	14.3
TOTALS:		**107**	**27.1**	**0**	**0.1**	**0**	**1.4**	**5.3**	**19.3**

DINNER-6:45 PM
FATS

FOOD ITEM	SERV.	CAL	CARBS	SAT	UNSAT	TRANS	PROTEIN	FIBER	SUGAR
Salad Dress. Red Wine Vin.	2 tbls.	85	7	1	3.5	0	0	0	4
Spinach/raw	3 cups	20	3	0	0	0	2	2	0
Broccoli/raw	1 Cup	25	4	0	0	0	3	3	1
Cucumber	1/4	30	5	0	0	0	0.5	2	0
Tomato	1/2 Md.	11	2.4	0.1	0.3	0	1.0	1.5	3.0
Roasted Turkey	56g	80	6	0.5	1.5	0	5	0	2
Spinach/cook	2/3 cup	30	3	0	0	0	2	2	0
Blk. eyed peas	½ cup	120	22	0	0	0	8	5	0
Brown Rice	¼ cup	170	36	0	1.5	0	4	2	0
TOTALS:		**571**	**88.4**	**6.1**	**6.8**	**0**	**25.5**	**17.5**	**10**

OTHER SNACKS

FOOD ITEM	SERV.	CAL	CARBS	SAT/UNSAT/TRANS (FATS)			PROTEIN	FIBER	SUGAR
Peanuts	116 g.	165	6	2	14	0	7	2	1
Sardines	92 g.	150	0	2	10	0	19	0	0
Graham Cr.	2 Cr.	130	11	0	1.5	0	1	0	4.4
TOTALS:		**445**	**17**	**4**	**25.5**	**0**	**27**	**2**	**5.4**

	CAL	CARBS	SAT/UNSAT/TRANS			PROTEIN	FIBER	SUGAR
TOTALS:	**2,471**	**2609***	**19.7**	**66.2**	**0**	**105.7**	**47.4**	**70.3****

*All carbs, with the exception of the chips, are unprocessed.
**Natural sugar, unlike added and artificial sugar, is accompanied with vitamins, minerals and fiber that slows down the insulin rush.

Note: I get out of bed and drink 3 cups of water every morning. I drink a cup of hot green tea every morning and consume at least 15-20 cups of water daily.

All numbers are in grams unless otherwise stated.

This is a light day of eating for me. My protein intake is usually much higher but I did not want to give you my workout nutrition plan because not everyone works out religiously.

As stated earlier, my purpose here is not to contend that this fuel plan is the gold standard for everyone. I'm sure there are unlimited plans that work for a variety of people. This is just an example of one way to self-monitor your eating and this is what has worked for me according to what I have experimented with from education to trial and error. This is also not all inclusive. I do have the occasional sweets and indulgences but not on a regular basis.

Summary: Abraham Maslow, American psychologist, placed self-actualization at the top of the pyramid of his hierarchy of human needs pyramid. This is finding your ultimate purpose and living in that. I believe you have a certain sense of peace and satisfaction when you are aligned with your true purpose. Some people spend their whole lives as understudies because they are auditioning for the wrong part. It is not enough just to be present. Most people want to contribute. This is the whole concept of nutrition investigation if you will. There is a unique chemistry that is you and the answer lies in education and paying attention to your unique signals. Your metabolism will thank you with good health and wellness. So in the interest of making a commitment to giving your body what it needs, let's take that one step—jump the broom, if you will—to true health and wellness. I have the perfect partner.

CHAPTER 7
Quality Nutrition Wedding Vows

t is now time for you to dedicate your life to quality nutrition and in turn to good health and wellness for the rest of your life.

Quality Nutrition Vows: Dearly Beloved

MINISTER:

Dearly beloved, we are gathered together here in the sight of God—and in the face of this company—to join together YOUR NAME in nutritional matrimony to QUALITY NUTRITION, which is commended to be healthy for all and therefore not by any to be entered into unadvisedly or lightly, but reverently, discreetly, advisedly, and solemnly. Into this holy estate these two persons present now come to be joined. If any person can show just cause why they may not be joined together, please speak now or forever hold your peace.

Quality nutrition is the union of human and the consumption of quality carbohydrates, fats, and protein in the right amounts in heart, body, and mind. It is intended for their wellness in life—and for the help and comfort given each other in prosperity and adversity. But more importantly, it is a means through which a stable and healthy environment may be attained.

Through quality nutrition, YOUR NAME and GOOD FOOD CHOICES make a commitment together to face life's disappointments, embrace their dreams, realize their hopes, and accept each other's failures. They will promise to each other to aspire to these ideals throughout their life together, through mutual understanding, openness, and sensitivity to each other.

We are here today, before God—because quality nutrition is one of his most sacred wishes—to witness the joining in quality nutrition of the two. This occasion marks the celebration of love and commitment with which they begin their life together. And now—through healthy food choices—joins you together in one of the healthiest bonds.

MINISTER:

This is a beginning and a continuation of their growth as individuals. With mutual care, respect, responsibility, and knowledge comes the affirmation of each one's own life happiness, growth, and freedom. With respect for individual boundaries comes the freedom to love unconditionally. Within the emotional safety of a loving relationship, the knowledge offered each other becomes the fertile soil for continued growth. With care and responsibility toward self and each other comes the potential for full and happy lives.

By gathering together all the wishes of happiness and the fondest hopes for GROOM'S NAME and BRIDE'S NAME from all present here, we assure them that our hearts are in tune with theirs. These moments are so meaningful to all of us, for "what greater thing is there for two human souls than to feel that they are joined together—to strengthen each other in all labor, to minister to each other in all sorrow, to share with each other in all gladness?"

This relationship stands for love, loyalty, honesty, and trust, but most of all for friendship. Before they knew love, they were friends, and it was this seed of friendship that is their destiny. Do not think that you can direct the course of love—for love, if it finds you worthy, shall direct you.

Marriage is an act of faith and a personal commitment as well as a moral and physical union between two people. Marriage has been described as the best and most important relationship that can exist between them. It is the construction of their love and trust into a single growing energy of spiritual life. It is a moral commitment that requires and deserves daily attention. Marriage should be a lifelong consecration of the ideal of loving kindness—backed with the will to make it last.

Exchange of Vows
MINISTER TO YOU:

Do you, YOUR NAME, take QUALITY NUTRITION to be your partner, to live together after the laws of good food choices in the holy estate of wellness? Will you love it, comfort it, honor and keep it in sickness and in health, for sweet, for sour, for bitter, for salt, in sadness and in joy, to cherish and continually bestow upon it your body's deepest devotion, forsaking all simple sugars, bad fats, and processed foods, and keep yourself only unto it as long as you both shall live?

I will.

MINISTER TO QUALITY NUTRITION:

Do you, QUALITY NUTRITION, take YOUR NAME to be your partner, to live together after laws of good food choices in the holy estate of matrimony? Will you love him or her, comfort him or her, honor and keep him or her in sickness and in health, for healthy digestion, for insulin sensitivity, for a healthy immune system, for proper weight management, for prevention of all diseases and the pursuit of the best health, to cherish and continually bestow upon him or her your deepest devotion, forsaking all bad nutrition, and keep yourself only unto him or her as long as you both shall live?

I will.

Pronouncement
MINISTER:

May you always share with each other the gifts of love. Be one in heart and in mind. May you always create a home together that puts in your hearts love, generosity, and kindness.

Inasmuch as YOUR NAME and QUALITY NUTRITION have consented together in marriage before this company of friends and family and have pledged their faith and declared their unity by exchanging vows, they are now joined.

You have pronounced yourselves life partners, but remember to always be each other's best friend.

What therefore you have put your heart and mind to, let no unhealthy trend or practice put asunder.

And so, by the power vested in you by the state of your mind and the willpower in your heart, you are now one. And may your days be good and long upon the earth.

You may now embrace quality nutrition.

SUMMARY: I'm pretty sure some will laugh at this little analogy. Some will find it a bit juvenile and some may be a little offended by the reference. The bottom line is that you have to stand for something or fall for anything. There is a high percentage of us who are commitment phobic—mostly men, and rightly so. Our health and wellness is nothing to be cavalier about or to be taken for granted. So whatever works for you: a contract on the refrigerator, Post-it notes around the office, the constant check-in from a trusted friend, or other method. The harsh reality could be a forced relationship with a well-intended but impersonal acquaintance—the doctor. Take some of the stress off his or her plate and save yourself some time and money in the process. They have too many other relationships to foster. Ladies, this can be viewed as your biological clock ticking. Men, have that midlife crisis now and skip the age-scheduled dilemma. We all can be in control of our health and wellness with the proper commitment to our knowledge and consumption of quality nutrition.

CONCLUSION

Throughout this journey we have explored the basic components of how to figure ourselves out. So many health-and-wellness companies and products make far-reaching claims and guarantees that categorize people into the one-size-fits-all category. Doctors and therapists treat symptoms, oftentimes not considering the origin of the condition. Big pharmaceutical companies maintain economic success off the progression of symptoms. Society is so transfixed on the outer appearance that it is blind to the reality of the basic needs of the organism from a biological perspective. I believe it is through education and personal investigation that we truly give ourselves the best chance to reach our highest quality-of-life potential. Real health and wellness can come only from the one who knows most about the body he or she has inherited. Yes, there are biological and chemical constants throughout the human body. Yes, we need to visit doctors because they have the knowledge and technology to give us basic checks and balances upon which we can now form a basis for self-care. But once the body receives macro- and micronutrients, the task becomes specific and unique to the individual on several levels. The chef uses most of the same ingredients used by novice cooks every day. The magic is in his or her unique way of blending portion, time, temperature, and other personal touches that transform those ingredients into a marketable final product. That magic took some time and trial and error to get things just right. Hopefully, you now have the ingredients to create your perfect final product. Relationships take time, trial and error to somewhat perfect. Take time to learn who you are-family reunion. Get smart on all micro and macronutrient properties and behaviors. Pay attention to how your system responds to the relationships you enter into and adjust as necessary. The knowledge of yourself and the energy that you meticulously ingest can foster a healthy and long-lasting relationship built on the qualities that you have proven are right for you. True love is out there and ready for you to embrace it.

REFERENCES

Joshua Rosenthal, "Integrative Nutrition": Greenleaf Book Group, 2007

Jennie Brand-Miller, PhD, Thomas M.S. Wolever, MD, PhD, Stephen Colagiuri, MD, Kaye Foster-Powell, M Nutr & Diet, "The New Glucose Revolution: The Authoritative Guide to the Glycemic Index-The dietary Solution to Permanent Weight Loss", Rodale, Inc, 2005

Dr. Barry Sears, "The Anti-Inflammation Zone: Reversing The Silent Epidemic That's Destroying Our Health", HarperCollins Publishing, 2005

Paul Insel, Don Ross, Kimberly McMahon, Melissa Bernstein, "Nutrition", Jones and Bartell Publishers, LLC., 2011

(http://nutritiondata.self.com/topics/glycemic-index)

(http://www.mindbodygreen.com/0-10339/5-things-you-need-to-know-about-your-blood-type.html)

(http://www.dadamo.com/txt/index.pl?1001)

GLOSSARY

Antibody: A protein used by the body to neutralize harmful substances in our bodies.

Antigen: Any substance that causes an immune system to produce antibodies against it.

Artificial Sweetener: A non-caloric substitute for sugar that is often more sweet, such as aspartame, acesulfame potassium, saccharin, alitame, and sucralose

Calorie: The energy needed to raise the temperature of 1 gram of water through 1 °C

Carbohydrate: Any of a large group of organic compounds occurring in foods and living tissues and including sugars, starch, and cellulose. They contain hydrogen and oxygen in the same ratio as water (2:1) and typically can be broken down to release energy in the animal body.

Cholesterol: A compound of the sterol type found in most body tissues, including the blood and the nerves. Cholesterol and its derivatives are important constituents of cell membranes and precursors of other steroid compounds, but high concentrations in the blood (mainly derived from animal fats in the diet) are thought to promote atherosclerosis.

Complex Carbohydrate: A polysaccharide (as starch or cellulose) consisting of usually hundreds or thousands of monosaccharide units; also : a food (as rice or pasta) composed primarily of such polysaccharides.

Craving: A powerful desire for something.

Fat: A natural oily or greasy substance occurring in animal bodies, especially when deposited as a layer under the skin or around certain organs.

Fatty Acid: A carboxylic acid consisting of a hydrocarbon chain and a terminal carboxyl group, especially any of those occurring as esters in fats and oils.

Fiber: Dietary material containing substances such as cellulose, lignin, and pectin, which are resistant to the action of digestive enzymes.

Free Fatty Acid: A carboxylic **acid** with a long aliphatic chain, which is either saturated or unsaturated.

Fructose: A hexose sugar found especially in honey and fruit.

Glucose: A simple sugar that is an important energy source in living organisms and is a component of many carbohydrates.

Glycemic Index: A system that ranks foods on a scale from 1 to 100 based on their effect on blood-sugar levels.

Glycemic Load: Calculated by multiplying the grams of available carbohydrate in the food times the food's GI and then dividing by 100.

Gout: A disease in which defective metabolism of uric acid causes arthritis, especially in the smaller bones of the feet, deposition of chalkstones, and episodes of acute pain.

Ghrelin: An enzyme produced by stomach lining cells that stimulates appetite.

High Density Lipoprotein (HDL): A lipoprotein that removes cholesterol from the blood and is associated with a reduced risk of atherosclerosis and heart disease.

Hormone: A regulatory substance produced in an organism and transported in tissue fluids such as blood or sap to stimulate specific cells or tissues into action.

Inflammation: A localized physical condition in which part of the body becomes reddened, swollen, hot, and often painful, especially as a reaction to injury or infection.

Insulin: A hormone produced in the pancreas by the islets of Langerhans that regulates the amount of glucose in the blood. The lack of insulin causes a form of diabetes.

Insulin Insensitivity: A pathological condition in which cells fail to respond normally to the hormone insulin. Also referred to as insulin resistance..

Insulin Sensitivity: A general phenomena in the body, and can be measured a few ways through studies. The pancreas (an organ that regulates blood sugar) secretes **insulin** in response to high blood sugar, and cells (like muscle or fat cells) can absorb blood sugar when stimulated by insulin.

Lactose: A sugar present in milk. It is a disaccharide containing glucose and galactose units.

Leptin: A protein produced by fatty tissue and believed to regulate fat storage in the body.

Low Density Lipoprotein (LDL): A microscopic blob that's made up of an outer rim of lipoprotein that surrounds a cholesterol center.

Metabolism: The chemical processes that occur within a living organism in order to maintain life.

Monosacharride: Any of the class of sugars (e.g., glucose) that cannot be hydrolyzed to give a simpler sugar.

Monounsaturated Fat: Fat molecules that have one unsaturated carbon bond in the molecule, this is also called a double bond. Oils that contain monounsaturated fats are typically liquid at room temperature but start to turn solid when chilled.

Natural Sweetener: Substances used to improve the palatability and shelf life of food products. Sugars occur naturally in many plant foods; we get most common sweeteners by processing these plants (such as agave cacti, maple trees, sugar cane, coconut palms, sugar beets and corn) to extract and condense the sugars.

Non-Alcoholic Fatty Liver Disease (NAFLD): The build up of extra fat in liver cells that is not caused by alcohol. It is normal for the liver to contain some fat. However, if more than 5% - 10% percent of the liver's weight is fat, then it is called a fatty liver (steatosis).

Omega-3 Fatty Acid: An unsaturated fatty acid of a kind occurring chiefly in fish oils, with three double bonds at particular positions in the hydrocarbon chain.

Photosynthesis: The process by which green plants and some other organisms use sunlight to synthesize foods from carbon dioxide and water. Photosynthesis in plants generally involves the green pigment chlorophyll and generates oxygen as a byproduct.

Polysaccharride: A carbohydrate (e.g., starch, cellulose, or glycogen) whose molecules consist of a number of sugar molecules bonded together.

Polyunsaturated Fat: Lipids in which the constituent hydrocarbon chain possesses two or more carbon–carbon double bonds. Polyunsaturated fat can be found mostly in nuts, seeds, fish, algae, leafy greens, and krill. "Unsaturated" refers to the fact that the molecules contain less than the maximum amount of hydrogen.

Protein: Any of a class of nitrogenous organic compounds that consist of large molecules composed of one or more long chains of amino acids and are an essential part of all living organisms, especially as structural components of body tissues such as muscle, hair, collagen, etc., and as enzymes and antibodies.

Satiation: To satisfy to the full; sate.

Saturated Fat: A fat that contains only saturated fatty acids, is solid at room temperature, and comes chiefly from animal food products. Some examples of saturated fat are butter, lard, meat fat, solid shortening, palm oil, and coconut oil. Saturated fat tends to raise the level of cholesterol in the blood.

Simple Carbohydrate: Sugars made of just one or two sugar molecules. They are the quickest source of energy, as they are very rapidly digested. Some food sources of simple carbohydrates: Table sugar.

Sodium: Sodium chloride or sodium bicarbonate present in or added to foods or beverages as seasoning or preservative.

Sugar: A sweet crystalline substance obtained from various plants, especially sugar cane and sugar beet, consisting essentially of sucrose, and used as a sweetener in food and drink.

Trans Fat: An unsaturated fatty acid of a type occurring in margarines and manufactured cooking oils as a result of the hydrogenation process, having a trans arrangement of the carbon atoms adjacent to its double bonds. Consumption of such acids is thought to increase the risk of atherosclerosis.

Unsaturated Fat: Fats or fatty acids that are liquid a room temperature. Unsaturated fats are derived from plants and some animals. They contain at least one double bond in their fatty acid chain. Conversely, a saturated fat has no double bonds meaning it is saturated with hydrogen atoms.

Water: A colorless, transparent, odorless, tasteless liquid that forms the seas, lakes, rivers, and rain and is the basis of the fluids of living organisms.

www.ingramcontent.com/pod-product-compliance
Lightning Source LLC
Chambersburg PA
CBHW060210290526
45789CB00003B/1224